Challenging Ideas in Psychiatric Nursing

Psychiatric nurses comprise the largest group of mental health professionals and the most divided. Ongoing preoccupations with the nature of mental illness, the relative efficacy of treatments and professional identity undermine calls for unity and divert attention away from the pressing needs of patients.

Challenging Ideas in Psychiatric Nursing arose out of the author's concern for the state of psychiatric nursing and its effect on patient care. Focusing on the basic assumptions which currently underpin education and practice, Liam Clarke calls into question the validity of 'holism' as an alternative knowledge base for nursing, the wholesale acceptance of Rogerian principles and leanings towards a reductionist approach. His book is an attempt to refocus attention on finding practical ways of helping the mentally ill to live in society rather than in conflict with it.

Challenging Ideas in Psychiatric Nursing will be an essential and thought-provoking read for nurses and other mental health professionals who want to develop as critical practitioners.

Liam Clarke is Lecturer in Mental Health at the University of Brighton at Falmer.

Challenging Ideas in Psychiatric Nursing

Liam Clarke

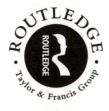

London and New York

First published 1999
by Routledge
11 New Fetter Lane, London EC4P 4EE

Simultaneously published in the USA and Canada
by Routledge
29 West 35th Street, New York, NY 10001

Routledge is an imprint of the Taylor & Francis Group

Typeset in Times by Routledge
Printed and bound in Great Britain by St Edmundsbury Press,
Bury St Edmunds, Suffolk

British Library Cataloguing in Publication Data
A catalogue record for this book is available from the British Library

Library of Congress Cataloging in Publication Data
Clarke, Liam, 1946–
Challenging ideas in psychiatric nursing/Liam Clarke.
Includes bibliographical references and index.
1. Psychiatric nursing. 2. Holistic nursing. I. Title.
[DNLM: 1. Psychiatric Nursing. 2. Holistic Nursing. WY 160 C598c
1999]
RC440.C537 1999
610.73´68–dc21
DNLM/DLC
for Library of Congress   98–32451

ISBN 0–415–18696–X (hbk)
ISBN 0–415–18697–8 (pbk)

For my wife
Johanna Clarke

Contents

Preface

This book is concerned with psychiatric nursing. I use this term, rather than mental health nursing, because many of the issues and controversies which concern this group of nurses arise from the nature of mental illness and the manner in which it has historically been responded to by psychiatry. As the book unfolds issues will arise which may be of some relevance to nurses generally and, of course, related professionals such as doctors, psychologists and social workers are welcome to speculate on the implications which this discussion might have for them.

At first sight the range of topics included in the book might appear daunting. However, a small number of themes organises these topics into what I believe to be the central concerns of psychiatric nurses today. A major theme is the evolution of holism and its connection with the influential theories of Carl Rogers. Holism has played a significant role in determining the nature of much current care. Its influence has been evident not only in psychological theories but also in current nurse education and its emphasis on health rather than illness. These aspects of the holistic influence are addressed in chapters 2, 3 and 9. Another theme of the book is the nature of psychiatric nursing. In chapters 7 and 8 I review specific counselling approaches and a certain kind of humanistic philosophy which have come to characterise psychiatric nursing for some. For others, the issues are not so clear cut and chapter 4 worries again at a timeless bone of contention in psychiatric nursing, namely custodialism versus the caring role. Chapter 5 looks at the fashionable theme of postmodernity. Whilst some might regard this chapter as a mere 'flight of fancy' it is important in respect of the comparative relevance of postmodernist 'theory' and the question of moral judgements in nursing. In addition, in chapter 6 I try to disentangle the emergence of some of these ideas and their continued relevance to a troubled nursing profession. Finally, in my opening and closing chapters I have tried to weave these topics into a tapestry which shows that there can be no resolution of what psychiatric nursing means without regard to a moral perspective which takes account of the patient's experience and the role of the carer in representing that experience to others. Such a perspective places the psychiatric nurse *outside* the usual concerns of professional practice: in effect, he or she may even oppose such practice on behalf of patients. At the same time, it is hoped that the reader will absorb the tension which runs through these chapters, especially where opposing viewpoints strive mightily for just such a professional evidence-based practice.

In order to impose a framework on the discussion the book sets out to find answers to a series of questions. The main question is one which has bewitched, bothered and bewildered nurse 'philosophers' for some time, namely 'what is nursing?', or more specifically for our purposes, 'what is psychiatric nursing?' Too many people rush to judgement on this, at times ending up in an abstract soup in which they flounder and sometimes drown. We shall proceed carefully, dutifully giving weight to various aspects of the arguments. This exploration invokes a range of issues which others have already examined in different contexts, but as nurses have not been conspicuous in their contribution to ideological, political or historical debates until recently, the presentation of some of these issues within a psychiatric nursing context may prove refreshing.

In asking 'what is psychiatric nursing?' it is anticipated that some of the answers which come about will relate to nursing as a whole. Recent developments in nursing generally, such as the tendency to equate nursing with this or that concept of caring, the stress on individualism, or the much vaunted entrance of nursing into the ranks of 'learned' professions are issues which affect all branches of the profession. We naturally shall concentrate on how psychiatric nursing relates to these developments so as to elicit differences as well as similarities between both arms of the profession. One warning before we start: the purpose of this book is to provide one point of view and not a balanced consideration of different or opposing positions. For example, it will be asserted that nursing of any kind cannot be a scientific discipline, in any normative sense of the word. However, this does not mean that in searching for answers, equal status will not be accorded other positions en route. It is high time that nurses came to conclusions about some things: we have been searching for a sense of 'who are we' and 'where are we going' for too long. Such lengthy inquiries are hardly problematic for most philosophical inquiry. However, their connection with practice places some obligation on nurses to declare themselves on some of the key issues.

Acknowledgements

Earlier versions of some of these chapters have appeared in journal form and I would like to acknowledge and thank the following for permission to utilise them here. Blackwell Science Ltd and the *Journal of Advanced Nursing* for permission to use material for chapter 5. *Nursing Times Research* (emap Healthcare) and the journal *Changes* for permission to use the respective papers which formed the basis for chapter 4. Editor Daniel Allen and *Mental Health Nursing* for the paper which now underpins chapter 7. And finally, the *British Journal of Psychotherapy*, in which some of the material in the book was first published.

Every effort was made to contact authors and copyright holders, but if proper acknowledgement has not been made, the copyright holder should contact the publishers.

1 Psychiatric nursing
Illusion and reality

Connections

Client care is central in discussing what psychiatric nursing is. The manner in which theories are used becomes important whatever the validity or otherwise of a particular theory. Let us examine this in relation to the question of science. Since the Enlightenment, we have grappled with two dimensions of science. One is the undoubted advances which (medical) sciences have brought to our understanding of the body and its ills. The second is the repeated abuses which science permits (for instance the gratuitous leucotomies of the 1950s and 1960s) and it is this second aspect which obliges us to look carefully at what people *do* with science. This particular discussion is apt in the light of recent calls (Gournay 1995; McFadyen and Vincent 1998) for psychiatric nurses to re-adopt a medical view of psychiatric disorder. That contention is refuted here by the simple counter-point that it is what nurses *do* with clients which matters rather than the rights or wrongs of any particular view. Psychiatry is a practical business and the theoretical basis of a treatment may not be pertinent. For example, few deny the efficacy of behaviour therapy for phobic disorders as opposed to psychoanalysis even if the latter seems 'made' for the high symbolism of the phobias. However, it hardly follows that behaviourism takes philosophical precedence over psychoanalysis as an account of human behaviour: clearly it does not. This disjunction between theory and action is actually a main plank in psychiatric history. Compare the way in which the assertions of R.D. Laing, produced during a period of high social unrest, exerted as much influence as his written work. As Joseph Berke remarked at the time (Clare 1996), 'Laing put the person back into the patient' and that is why he made a difference. After him, the stigmatising did not stop but it was now easily seen for the smear tactic it was. Today, Laing's anti-psychiatry stands accused of naïvety; his supposed unwillingness to engage with the biological data is seen as a mistake. This misses the point, however, which is that irrespective of their biology, schizophrenic patients (by whatever name) were asking to be recognised as people and Laing responded appropriately.

What reductionism in science can do is further delineate the neurological correlates of schizophrenia and other physical states. What nurses must do is guard against that degeneration by which biological/genetic models lead – as indisputably they did in the past – to mental illness being seen as inborn and irredeemable to the extent that patients become undervalued as people. When psychiatric drugs fail to work – even their strongest advocates acknowledge that failures occur – there is a noticeable withering away of psychologists and psychiatrists from the social world of schizophrenic patients and their nurses. It is at this juncture that psychiatric nurses can enter the social worlds of schizophrenic people, engaging their desires, hopes and ambitions.

Genetic and technological investigations are important in that they may ultimately provide predictive clues to the likelihood of schizophrenia in the new-born. However, the nurse's role is not to embrace 'the new genetics' but, working in tandem with schizophrenic people, to judge its worth relative to the overall quality of living which schizophrenic people *currently* enjoy.

Hippocrates states: 'It is more important to know what sort of patient has a disease than what sort of disease a patient has' (in Lloyd 1970). In the light of this, asking the question 'what is psychiatric nursing?' can allow us at least to say what it is not. It is not, for instance, about the theoretical correctness of scientific as opposed to experiential concepts of mental illness. By experiential concepts I mean any account which has as a part of its description the narratives of the person with the presumed condition. Rather, it is more concerned with interventions which take the form of social engagements with patients. It may seek an understanding of genetics, biochemistry, structural functionalism (to pick just one sociological concept) or even Rogerian therapy but only insofar as these *inform*, not define, the way in which one works with clients. This is, of course, not something about which all psychiatric nurses necessarily agree and, as we have observed, the 1990s has seen the re-awakening, in some circles, of technologically inspired attempts to define schizophrenia in biological terms, and to revive psychiatric nursing as a supportive agency within a dominant biomedical culture. Yet, to risk overstating the point, it is an historical 'truth' grounded in the testimony of those who were there (Martin 1984) that the asylum/hospital conditions which directly stemmed from medical constructs of illness and its treatment led inexorably to the doldrums of institutionalised nursing. This was a nursing comprised of hierarchies, rules, uniforms, the omnipotence of doctors, an obsession with illness and, especially, the 'death by boredom' of shift systems. There existed a slavish obedience to received ideas, especially within nurse training departments, whereby patients simply withered on the vine of concepts of chronic illness. In far too many cases these attitudes led to a slippage into abuse and neglect.

This sort of nursing practice, incapable of dealing with patients outside medical constructs, persisted within such settings until as recently as fifteen years ago. The issue is therefore about how nurses, who do not themselves play a large part in the development of medico-psychiatric constructs, interpret those constructs in delivering care to the patient and the extent to which they allow their actions to be governed by them. An uncritical acceptance of illness models leads to beliefs about incomplete recoverability and it is this kind of thinking which also fosters custodialism and despair.

The new technocracy of care

Recently, whilst reviewing a paper (Gournay and Brooking 1994) with a view to discovering something about its methods and design, it became apparent that the paper's quantitative methodology, whilst being described in terms of its investigative merits, was in addition being proselytised as a superior approach to research. It seemed that a sub-textual propaganda was afoot. From my initial concern with methodology I became fascinated by the furtive deployment of language against qualitative studies which, according to this paper, were failing in their refusal to genuflect before the high altar of statistics.

The paper addressed various aspects of community psychiatric nursing. It described the random assignment of groups of clients to different thera-peutic conditions and outlined the different client outcomes for these conditions, some surprising and some not. However, as the paper proceeded, it began to display a progressive displeasure that some Community Psychiatric Nurses (CPNS) were describing their work as 'counselling'. The paper made no attempt to find out what they might have meant by this but concentrated instead on the absence of controlled trials in support of coun-selling effectiveness. Surprisingly, in the absence of such trials, the authors conclude anyway that counselling appears not to be effective (1994: 236). This is quite a neat shift coming as it does from psychiatric writers who would appear to pride themselves on specificity, measurement and control: for, in effect, they correlate the absence of controlled studies with assump-tions about the effectiveness of that which has not been studied. Absence of evidence, in other words, becomes evidence of inefficacy. This paper is an example, par excellence, of what Hanfling (1978) calls a 'science has shown' argument, or to put this another way, discourse which seeks to show that scientific discoveries are as irresistible as progress itself.

The literature shows a growing interest in controlled trials of the 'experi-mental science' type and it is indeed remarkable how more and more psychiatric nurse researchers have adopted such experimentation without questioning its relevance to analysing patient relationships. What this sort of scientism ignores is the absence of any necessary connection between validity and fact. Simplistically, it impugns truths arrived at by different (that is, non-quantitative) means. Yet it is important to recognise that this re-colonisation of psychiatric nursing as a medico-scientific concern is itself a value-laden exercise. It has as one of its determinants a desire to take psychi-atric nursing away from concepts of democratic practice where *everyone's* voice would merit attention and to re-orient it towards precepts which are objective and measurable. If we are to contradict this scientism then we need briefly to look at how science works.

The appliance of science

Most applied scientists operate within a conventional mode of science, working out problems and seeking solutions to questions of acknowledged significance. They rarely venture near the indeterminacy of the 'new physics' nor do they seek to concurrently disprove that which they are actively researching. Hugh Dudley (1996), in this instance, makes a distinction between science and scientific advance, by which he means that whilst most scientists work within conventional boundaries of testing their hypotheses, when scientific conclusions arrived at logically are at odds with underlying theory, they will remain sceptical and be prepared to shift their ground. They will balance 'the facts' against theory. What they will not do is use 'the latest findings' as a battering ram against colleagues who choose to differ and, of course, from a Popperian perspective, this would be a decidedly unscientific thing to do. The Gournay/Brooking paper, for example, masquerades as dispassionate writing, whilst implicitly condemning research which either relies on literary discourses or patients' narratives of their experiences. One would expect truly objective papers to concentrate on the significance of what leaves the laboratory bench, letting the findings speak for themselves, and it is therefore surprising to find that they are as politically motivated as any other kind of work. Although the full implications of their rhetoric are not spelt out, it does appear to hold that medical concepts of illness are fundamental: people have illnesses; these illnesses require treatments which can either be physical treatments or of a type which rely only minimally on human discourse and so, by their nature, produce measurable outcomes. The twin branches of psychoanalytic and humanistic therapies are rejected.

How is psychiatric nursing defined under these conditions? In addition to the provision of treatments it may also be about connecting nursing actions to beliefs about 'enduring and serious' mental illness with diminishing emphasis on 'problems' that are difficult to classify as illnesses. Interventions requiring lengthy contact time or the kind of interactive relationships which are difficult to quantify because they are unique will be sidelined. In short only that nursing which can produce evidence for what it does – specifying interventions and outcomes discretely – may be deemed worthy of inclusion.

Defining nursing

My purpose is not to attack approaches based on concepts of illness nor to castigate the kinds of research and treatments they appear to warrant. Rather my challenge to those who espouse these approaches, is that they identify the bits which comprise *nursing* and defend their position within a nursing context. The problem for them is that in using serious and enduring illness as a starting point, interventions are either going to be cognitive–behaviourist in nature, thus edging nursing towards a psychological mode of practice, or they are going to be of a nature which will return nurses to the role of interminable second-fiddle to a medical speciality which enduringly controls diagnosis and prescription. In fact, the positions spearheaded by writers such as Gournay (1995) and Ritter (1997) are only viable in connection with medicine although they might point to initiatives such as the Thorn Programme (Gamble 1995) to refute this. Whilst anything that helps disabled people is to be welcomed, I am persuaded that Thorn programmes are as valuable to professional ascendancy as they are to patient care. An analogy can be made here with the introduction of phenothiazine drugs in the 1950s whereby these too heralded such high optimism that a feedback loop occurred in which higher and higher dosages of them were given. Since one imagines that the aim of pharmacology is to get the greatest benefit from the lowest dosage of a given drug it is surprising how rare this has been in psychiatry where drugs have often been used excessively and sometimes punitively (Breggin 1993). The same applies to Thorn where a modest package of psycho-social interventions has become regarded as a veritable 'magic bullet', which it is not. What Thorn does allow are interventions capable of producing measurable outcomes with schizophrenic patients, the unacknowledged caveat being that observable improvements in socially deprived schizophrenic patients within short time periods are not difficult to achieve anyway.

What Thorn fails to take account of is the person's right to refuse such treatment. Indeed the problem with 'packages' like this is their inability to recognise the intransigent nature of chosen lifestyles as well as their tendency to respond to refusals of treatment in ways which iron out the possible complexities involved rather than engage with them. The role which the unconscious life might play in refusing help or even in courting despair is anathema. Similarly, the manner in which some people find comfort in drifting into vagrancy is inexplicable other than as some 'idiosyncratic' choice. It is therefore debatable whether Thorn, or anything like it, could bring about long-term change and even more questionable whether it could provide a substitute for the necessary social and political redress of injustices visited on psychotic people.

Thorn's defenders point to the 'evidence' of its success and use this in turn as a further endorsement of the randomised control method. Gournay, for example, states that 'those who are responsible for funding projects and making public policy view such trials as the ultimate test. Mental health nursing should ignore this method at its peril.' (This in itself is an interesting 'disclosure' of who nurses should see as their significant audience.) The problem with controlled analysis, however, is that its subject rarely extends beyond single items of behaviour and is usually cleansed of both individual experience and psycho-social influences such that any explanatory power which these might have is lost. In addition, quantitative studies take very little account of the narratives of their subjects (something on which much of physical medicine relies). What this leaves, in effect, is a definition of nursing that does not admit quality of interactions as a primary element and this has, intuitively, an odd quality to it: there is a feeling that nursing ought to be synonymous with interactions. Surely the proper focus of nursing is to acknowledge the psycho-social complexities of living rather than to engage in the practice of deciphering people so as to be in a better position to treat their illnesses.

Spelling it out

A particular feature endemic to much nursing discourse is a peculiar resolution not to spell out its terms, and the question of 'serious mental illness' is a case in point. There is rarely provided any rule or category by which to define 'seriousness'. Typically it is linked to 'enduring' and the clear impression conveyed is that we are dealing with schizophrenia (Brooker and Repper 1998). However, this still begs the question, what is meant by 'serious'? Can there be serious cases which are not enduring? And if so, serious to whom: the medical profession, patients, relatives or nurses? From the perspective of patients and their families seriousness may reside in the experience of illness rather than in considerations of diagnosis, hospitalisation, cost and so on. In a major text (Brooker and Repper 1998: 9) there occurs a frank confession of inability to define the terminology: 'Mental health problems will always pose dilemmas, so it is perhaps unsurprising that for the purposes of this book, we have not prescribed any particular definition.' Also, the quantitative position is essentially economic in nature, conscious of government provision and with a focus on the problem of schizophrenia as an epidemiological event. This position tries to be neutral, even uninterested, in how schizophrenia might be experienced other than as a neurological phenomenon.

Testing times

It was R.D. Laing who observed that you could learn all that there is to know about schizophrenia and still not know anything about a particular schizophrenic. This says something about the importance of recognising different kinds of knowledge and their application. Whilst some seek a form of knowledge about mental health which permits generalisations to be made, others care about little beyond individuals (whom they see as unique anyway) and so are content with a knowledge that is virtually untestable because embedded in the experiences of those concerned. As Rogers and Pilgrim (1996) observe, whilst epidemiological studies can provide data for the formulation of policies about the organisation and delivery of health care, questions concerning the epistemology of psychiatry and problems of legitimising psychiatric theory or psychiatric nursing practice are beyond their scope.

It is indeed foolish to believe that we are reaching a safe plateau from which to expound on the nature of mental illness with conviction. The lack of evidence for such 'convictions' is seen in the reliance on emotivism and 'persuader language' which is invariably present in scientistic writing:

> Although biological research has been proceeding at a breathtaking rate, our knowledge concerning the biological aetiological variables is far from complete.
>
> (Gournay 1997: 227)

The implication is that we are heading towards completion, indeed that we are *almost there*. By phrasing it like this, the notion of our knowledge in this area being actually meagre is avoided. In addition, a 'modesty angle' is built into the writing, the acknowledgement of 'not *quite* being there' clearly an effort at wooing the reader to the side of reasonableness and rationality. Indeed, this 'beginning to gel', this endless 'on the brink', 'imminent discovery' verbiage is really the hallmark of self-doubt and obfuscation.

In his earlier paper, Gournay (1995) had referred to growing knowledge in PET scan search as vast: longitudinal studies using brain imaging techniques plus genetic studies had, he insisted, 'revolutionised our understanding of a range of ideas'. We may well ask, how? In my view, we are no closer to understanding schizophrenia than we were thirty years ago. The argument that 'schizophrenia is best viewed as a group of disorders caused by abnormalities in brain development' (Gournay 1995: 8) is based on a primitive concept of genetics which leaves aside social and cultural aspects of the topic. It is an exceptionally queer form of nursing which adopts this view and constant use of the language of abnormality, disorder, illness and 'serious and enduring' is good evidence of the neglect of a nursing dimension in this approach.

What nursing is

The frantic search for a rationale for nursing proceeds apace and with hardly a passing glance at the work of psychiatric nurses. This is ironic given the extent to which both mental health nursing in Britain and the burgeoning nursing philosophies from America have been influenced by humanistic psychology and especially the work of Carl Rogers. Yet whatever unites or divides these philosophies, it is the desire for a non-medical identity which has provoked organisational and conceptual changes in modern British nursing. As we saw in the Hippocrates quote (above), the idea that there is more to people than just their illnesses is not new. What *is* new is the determination to take this idea literally and to then build a professional nursing role upon it.

There are significant differences between the kinds of debates which have fuelled the various branches of nursing but, to the limited extent that they have taken place, debates in psychiatric nursing have ultimately boiled down to questions about the nature of mental illness. It is important to re-emphasise that the real issue for nurses is about being less concerned with the theoretical correctness of definitions and more conscious of the moral worth which society places on affected individuals with the resultant question of how nurses might best help these individuals have a 'good life'. Questions of aetiology, brain scanning, cognitive function, pharmacology and biochemistry may be more intellectually respectable but they detract from the central issue of how best to enable people to live a reasonable life in terms which *they* see as reasonable and right. This, in my view, denotes illness as but one element to be considered (and not necessarily the most important element) in an overall approach to working through problems in the lives of mentally ill people.

Searching

On the trail of what a psychiatric nurse might be, Philip Barker allows that nurses complement the care given by doctors but that, in addition, they possess a quality of spiritual healing and that it is their handling of this 'psychic healing' dimension which distinguishes them from others. Barker is quite blunt about this: 'My belief is that psychiatric nursing is a spiritual activity' (1997: 319).

What, however, would this mean in practice? What might nurses 'do' as a function of their spirituality? For Barker, this is 'the question I am least confident about asking' (1997: 319). Unsurprisingly so far, apart from saying that the answer lies between the relationship of patient and nurse, little more is added. The patient's narrative, of course, is an important tool of recovery for both patient and nurse; both are empowered by their relationship. Patients are encouraged to 're-author their feelings', see their lives in a different way and so achieve a degree of healing. There is a point of connection here with the 'Hearing Voices Network' (Baker 1995) who advocate acknowledging voices so as to try and impose a measure of control over them. Other than that, it becomes difficult to see how Barker's position offers anything over and above, let's say, a typical Rogerian perspective which stresses the idea of the therapeutic journey, a self-enlightening exercise that runs the risk of being seen as idiosyncratic or esoteric. The latter seems not to phase its proponents but, of course, why should it, since by definition it celebrates individuality whilst rejecting generalisations about people.

It could be that, ultimately, this is what a theory of nursing will become: a resigned acceptance of essentially unique encounters between nurses and patients, individual renditions of problems and ills against a background of the basic humanities which define our culture. Certainly, it has not been possible to concoct a definition to which a majority (of nurses) could subscribe and the endless models and frameworks proposed, entertained and then abandoned are testimony to the mystery which lies at the heart of nursing. Hence there has been a rush by some to assume the mantle of physical sciences and medicalisation because the latter provides not just a delusion of scientific respectability but also an escape route from what might be seen as extremely dubious talk about spirituality.

The community

One measure of the heterogeneity of community psychiatric nursing is that most CPNs have not formally prepared for their task. The permutations of CPN practice have been reviewed elsewhere (Pollock 1989; Morrall 1994) and need not detain us. What is of interest, however, is that this sub-group which purports to be a speciality within psychiatric nursing is really a series of indeterminate undertakings. One of these undertakings however – a penchant for counselling people with 'problems in living' – is seen by some as constituting a neglect of those with serious and enduring illness. Community psychiatric nursing, says Peter Morrall (1994), ought to be about 'policing the mad' and others likewise have campaigned for community nurses to work with psychotic clients. All told, CPNs have seen their speciality constantly eroded, and if not quite the butt of societal displeasure in the way that social workers can be they are attacked on grounds of wearing themselves thin on the backs of what are called 'the worried well'. A range of factors have led to the current confusion of community psychiatric nurses, two of which will be explored here: the development of the concept of 'mental health nurses' and the movement of patients from hospital to community. These will be discussed against the background of the charge that community nurses have been working with the wrong client groups.

One recommendation of the Mental Health Nursing Review Team (1994) was that all psychiatric nurses – whether in the community or hospital based – be awarded the title 'mental health nurse'. This is quite astonishing for whatever chance one might have of defining mental illness, defining mental health (with its implications of normality/abnormality overlap) would be a formidable task indeed. In general, studies of CPN practice (Morrall 1994; Pollock 1989; Warner 1997) show a picture of great confusion and happenstance, a picture which is not helped by widespread scepticism about community care for mentally unwell people (Bowers 1997). Certainly, no country isolated its 'mad' as efficiently as did the English Victorians and one could hardly have expected any reversal of this to be easy. Another more likely reason for CPNs lacking a coherent theoretical stance is the range of their responsibilities and the 'catch-all' response position which this puts them in. Something of this diversity is reflected in the kinds of research which they undertake. On the one hand, there is a regular 'head count' exercise: the 'quinquennial national survey' (Brooker and White 1998), which tries to identify demographic shifts in CPN practice. Then, there are reported those infrequent but influential 'randomised control trials'. (These are a little dubious even on their own terms partly due to questionable samples but also their inability to account for psychosocial factors which attend most forms of CPN interventions.) Lastly, there are studies which question the role of community psychiatric nursing usually on the basis of preformed notions of what mental illness is and/or how it should be controlled.

Something which unites all of these studies is that they are carried out by what Tony Gillam (1995: 49) calls 'a hard nosed mob of professional researchers'. This is exemplified by a well-known series of books (Brooker and White 1990, 1993, 1995) in which a total of 59 chapters represented but eight contributions by practitioners. Such a theory–practice divide is disquieting amongst a relatively new branch of nursing which might have been expected to learn from the divisions of the past.

Of course, much of this discussion assumes the existence of a relatively straightforward CPN service 'out there' but as Ross *et al.* (1998) point out, the word 'community' is problematic in terms of what it means to different people and groups. The term 'psychiatric' is equally loaded with ideological connotations. Therefore, considering that the word 'nurse' is the most problematic of all, it is not difficult to see that any analysis of community psychiatric nursing must deal with the potential meanings to which these words give rise. I have mentioned that the humanistic and mystical fraternities in nursing are relatively content with semantic confusion since their focus is on inner experiencing anyway: they take it as read that categories are unhelpful (the DSM IV (1994) is seen by them as a mechanical delusion), a means of imposing order on recalcitrant behaviour. The opposing view, naturally, sees the DSM IV as 'a great improvement on taxonomy' (Gournay 1995) while at the same time acknowledging the difficulty of finding 'pure experimental groups' on which to test its treatments. For some, this heterogeneity in community nursing represents a healthy willingness to debate issues, to approach patients' problems in different ways. The quandary, if there is one, is that different groups appear to be talking about different things. One group has ceased to ask about the meaning of, let's say, schizophrenia having concluded that it is a brain disorder whilst another persists in holding to a concept of mind as something which is of a higher (or at least another) order of reasoning and experience.

Size

Size is a factor in any nursing discussion: numbers play their part. The sheer size of the nursing fraternity almost inevitably leads to division. Interestingly, only about 20 per cent of psychiatric nurses have ever worked in the community. The majority continue to occupy positions in treatment centres of one sort or another. Again, this poses the question of what is meant by the community. For instance, it is meaningless to refer to units (often former hospital wards) which nowadays operate from high street addresses as 'the

community' since many of these continue to operate within a medical orientation which hardly differs from its hospital antecedents. The capacity of these
units to mop up large numbers of patients is, however, nowhere as great as
the old hospital/asylums. Whereas, before the demise of the asylums, the
work of CPNs could indeed develop along psycho-therapeutic lines given
that psychotic patients were remorselessly hospitalised, this picture would
change with the closure of the hospitals and the re-emergence into the
community of significant numbers of schizophrenic patients. The needs of
these post-asylum patients extend beyond that which nurses operating
within a psycho-therapeutic orientation can reasonably meet. What is now
required by these patients is a social framework capable of providing reasonable options about how best to live their lives whilst assuring them of the
means to do it. Brooker and White's latest (1998) quinquennial study has
indeed discovered a shift by CPNs back towards working with people with
schizophrenia. Whether this has resulted from actual demand brought about
by hospital closures or is a reflection of the criticism that CPNs were failing
these patients is, however, difficult to say.

Fashions change

It has become fashionable to play down the possible effects of socialisation
on human behaviour in preference for DNA and other explanations of
human motivation. Time and again the media relate discoveries of genes
which explain this and genes which explain that. There are now genes for IQ,
homosexuality, alcoholism and even criminality. Rose notes (1998: 20) that,
according to Daniel Koshland (former editor of the prestigious *Science*),
there may even be a gene for homelessness.

Much of the salesmanship of scientism depends on similar fallacious
appeals to the mystique of 'the new genetics'. I referred earlier to 'persuader
language', devious attempts to win people over by employing 'cheaply
seductive dichotomies' of nature versus nurture (Rose 1998). Whereas there
is occasionally tacked on a 'sadly we do not yet know' apologia, this hardly
diminishes the facile assertion that ultimately science will answer all questions about human life.

Whatever the philosophical rightness of what science can or cannot do,
this is a good place to restate that this is not what nurses should be asking.
Much may be gained in employing a genetic or biochemical explanation for
human behaviour both in terms of prevention and physical treatments.
However, the latter have been significantly overrated even if beneficial to
particular individuals. Biological/genetic models have the effect of over-
emphasising medical perspectives and diverting inquiry (and funding) away
from social constructions of mental distress.

From the 1960s, a pseudo-liberal agenda had defined social constructions
of mental illness as warmer, less harsh than medical approaches with their
drugs, electric treatment and so on. Such constructions attained a high moral

ground, apparently lacking any awareness of their dependent position within overall egalitarian trends of this century. The point about contemporary resurrections of schizophrenia as a product of neuropathology (Andreasen 1985; Crow 1993), is that these are social constructions too. That their polemic is couched in a language of chemistry and technology appears to imbue them with an over-arching authority but this is undeserved. Laying ideas upon a bed of chemistry may lend a veneer of scientific respectability to debate. Indeed, attributing semantic meanings to empirical findings can exceed what these findings actually support. Churchland (1988) notes that definitions and 'constructions of meaning' which precede empirical work are misplaced. The science bench, she affirms, will evolve its own amplifications or replacements of current definitions. One wishes that positivist nurses would take note of this and allow their findings a degree or two of independence from the excessive proselytising with which they have surrounded them so far. Mundt and Spitzer (1993) point out that whereas in the 1950s and 1960s proponents of interpretative approaches probably overstated their case in terms of generality and applicability, it is the natural sciences which currently do this. Actually, to claim that improved medical technology is salient to nurses is cavalier. Rather, nurses inhabit the social worlds of schizophrenic people with their concerns about social survival and well-being and it is here that nurses are likely to be of assistance. Whilst bio-technology may eventually *prevent* forms of schizophrenia, it remains of doubtful benefit to current sufferers.

Institution or community

Whilst calls for a re-medicalisation of schizophrenia seek to solicit links with hospital nurses, in general these nurses are inclined to play down theoretical formulations (Caudill 1958; Davis 1981; White 1985; Clarke 1991). Current discussions have evolved around CPNs possibly because their practice seemed to part company with biological concepts of illness, moving instead towards social constructions (Pollock 1989; Barker *et al.* 1998). There developed a false impression of psychiatric nursing having moved away from medical constructs when in truth only some CPNs had done this. However, it was this perception coupled with observed changes in the provision of care which provoked the critique of working with 'the worried well'.

It is hardly surprising that in an age of reverence for 'can do' philosophies, attempts by the Right to audit psychiatric nursing should emerge. We have seen, particularly in the USA, the rise of didactic therapies such as ordeal or reality therapy (Glasser 1975), rational emotive therapy (Ellis 1962), neuro-linguistic programming (Bandler and Grinder 1979) and so forth; curious amalgams of advice, admonition and control. In Britain, Garth Wood, a General Practitioner, propagates moral therapy and in his book *The Myth of Neurosis* (1983), lambastes all who stray outside a tightly contrived band of psychoses and clinical neuroses. Curiously, current criticisms from within nursing (Ward 1994; Gournay and Beadsmore 1995) have not mined this vein of moral contempt for those whose problems do not amount to 'real illness'. In fact, much of the nursing debate proceeds as if vacuumed off from contemporary political/moral nostrums about eligibility, self-help, dependence and welfare (Darcy 1994). However, people with so-called minor or 'neurotic' conditions are no less terrorised by them as people with schizophrenia.

Human distress is its own barometer and illness categories are no measure of misery. Some people with schizophrenia lead reasonable, productive lives. Others experience problems in living and whilst they may lack disturbances of affect or cognition, they may nevertheless come to experience serious social breakdown, loss of esteem or control and even suicide. One expression of this is the large number of young people who present at A&E departments following acts of self-mutilation. It has become commonplace for these patients to be treated with contempt by casualty staff and they frequently complain of rejection and humiliation especially if they have a history of asking for help (see Clarke and Whittaker 1998). This well-established A&E phenomenon (Pembroke 1991) suggests a basic lack of sympathy for complaints which are perceived by nursing staff as minor or trivial. May and Kelly (1982) have similarly shown how such rejection can occur within psychiatric settings where some patients' 'nuisance value' is offset by their schizophrenia as opposed to those whose culpability is enhanced by their psychopathy. It can be seen as such that differences in responding to different groups of patients is already an established phenomenon in nursing care. What matters is that whatever the rationale of rationing, nurses need to explain the moral background which informs particular decisions.

Some years ago when a general hospital announced cessation of resuscitation for the over-65s, a newspaper cartoon showed a terrified old man sitting before an imperious hospital almoner and the caption underneath read 'I'm only sixty four: honestly, I'm just sixty four.' Rationing care diminishes the dignity of the human spirit. It is a shameful exercise because according to Brooker and White (1998) the number of CPNs stands at about 9,500 which is by no means a large number given the shut down of much of the hospital provision. It is shameful because rather than demand a modest increase of ten or fifteen per cent more CPNS, what we are presented with is a campaign which seeks to ensure cover for some groups (serious and enduring) by means of the concerted neglect of others (the so-called 'worried well').

No easy answers

A central question for nurses is how to define those rights and dignities which should lie at the heart of every human encounter. In September 1957, Thomas Percival Rees, Superintendent of Warlingham Park Hospital, called for a return to the age-old values of respect, dignity and civility for patients:

everything else he believed, all progress, would flow from this. Today it is acknowledged (sometimes grudgingly) that post-1950s changes in the lives of patients resulted from the kinds of social forces epitomised by Rees' address and not from the so-called 'phenothiazine revolution' (Henderson and Gillespie 1956). In fact the introduction of these drugs was but a part of changes which were already underway such as the spread of 'the open door movement' and the emergence of small numbers of therapeutic communities (Jones 1982; Clarke 1994).

In the 1960s, there arose a deeper, more intellectual, critique of psychiatric practice deriving inspiration from philosophically radical, especially continental, sources. In Britain, this movement was led by R.D. Laing who achieved some prominence amongst the scientific, artistic and wider community. His concepts of illness rarely permeated everyday practice, other than a small number of private units of which the best known was Kingsley Hall (Clay 1996). In respect of the NHS, a unit called Villa 21 did open at Shenley hospital, St Albans, but was peremptorily closed (Cooper 1970). (For a dramatic reconstruction – including footage shot at Villa 21 – of this period in psychiatric history see Ken Loach's 1971 fictional film *Family Life*.) Conventional psychiatry appeared to go its own way, embarrassed by Laing, and increasingly tongue-tied in trying to account for some of its physical treatments and the problem of explaining why they so frequently needed to be forced on patients. Of course psychiatry had always been uneasy about the 'limitations' of its armamentarium: from Mason Cox (1896) who suspended patients in cages rotating one hundred times a minute (many of them immediately asserted their recovery) to Manfred Sakel (1938) who comatosed schizophrenics with insulin, there has been hydrotherapy, mosquito therapy, electric therapy, carbon dioxide therapy, dialysis and narcosis therapy and, of course, chemotherapy. What unites these 'therapies' is an enduring commitment to finding something to do with patients coupled necessarily with the belief that the discovery of a curative physical treatment is imminent (Horrobin 1980; Macdonald and Merritt 1996). Of course, without this constant searching progress would stop and it is fitting to wish laboratory studies well. Having said this, if anything comes from the history of physical treatments in psychiatry it must surely be a healthy scepticism although you would hardly notice it in the manner by which most psychiatric nurses remain favourably disposed towards physical treatments. Whilst this latter statement might (rightly) raise some eyebrows amongst community psychiatric nurses we can be quite confident about its truth for the majority who continue to work in in-patient treatment settings. The palpable lack of interest shown by researchers in these nurses needs to be accounted for.

The CPNs

The brunt of the critique against working with 'less seriously ill people' has been aimed at CPNs. Yet, CPNs, we have noted, are a disparate collection of practitioners and the predilection of some for working with neurotic as opposed to psychotic patients seems to have come about as much through opportunity as through any concerted shift in ideology or theory of practice. However, in order to push home the point about their neglect of seriously ill patients their critics had to sidestep the fact that CPNs are a small minority (of psychiatric nurses) as well as the troublesome issue of the majority of institutional nurses never having abandoned a medical epistemology in the first place, an epistemology which these critics now sought to re-introduce!

The background to these debates was the shifting emphasis of care from old institutional settings to 'the community' and the political dynamite of disoriented schizophrenic patients behaving badly and causing offence. The CPN service, having evolved with ample hospital backup, was hardly prepared for the sudden discharge of psychiatric patients on to their doorsteps, an event which resulted in a kind of moral panic and confusion. Immediately CPNs became vulnerable to pressure from the medically inclined amongst them to re-adopt a strategy of pathology-based manage-ment. In general this has resulted in a classic nursing acquiescence to a higher (this time political) power and specifically an inability to combat cost-driven police functions introduced after some well-publicised murders by psychiatric patients.

There is a more balanced view. Bowers (1997), for example, discusses a range of options, two of which he identifies as conferring a unique status on practising nurses: a) identification with users and b) politicising interventions on user's behalf. However, he then discounts the importance of these on the grounds of a post-Thatcher demoralisation of CPNs on the one hand and the lack of a coherent user perspective on the other. These are fair points although it is because users' views differ, it is because they shout with indi-vidual voices that their 'position' is attractive.

Taking off

There is no universally agreed definition of what psychiatric nursing is although brave hearts are quick to say what it ought to be. This problem of a clear-cut identity is part of the difficulty in setting a financial rate for nurses. If they are a profession of equal standing to others then why are their salaries significantly lower? At a time when the British government is proposing to question the preparation and role of nurses in what sense can we assert that nursings' aspirations are free from outside interference? To what extent is autonomous practice possible? In July 1998 the *Nursing Times* reported a nurse's complaint that she would not be welcome back at her hospital unless she made the tea for medical staff. It needed a visit by this nurse to the media to force the hospital to change its mind. This is more than an isolated incident and there are no shortage of clashes whenever nurses are motivated by concepts of professional status and especially ethical considerations about what constitutes the best care. Equally other nurses (perhaps the majority) are motivated by occupational issues especially in respect of how they perceive managerial and/or administrative requirements. As Richardson reports (1998: 18), attitudes towards professional practice differ markedly between nursing and medicine. Unlike their medical counterpart nurses are seemingly unwilling to rely on professional rationales for their actions, opting instead for occupational/managerial justifications.

Management and profession may not mix. Indeed nursing management and nurses may have entirely different agendas, witness the enthusiastic and derogatory manner (Hart 1994) in which grading systems were implemented and the difficulties which many nurses had in articulating their professional role. Says Richardson (1998 :18):

> Unless the culture of nursing management alters, there will be no way that the profession can go forward, become autonomous and take on more areas of responsibility – with the attendant risks.

Indeed, so much that occurs in nursing may be problematic especially where decisions continue to be taken in politicised contexts. A few years ago I conducted a series of observations (Clarke 1996) within forensic psychiatric units and I thought that the different forces which these units represented were an apt microcosm for the problems of psychiatric nursing generally. I became party to serious in-fighting between two groups of nurses on the very question of the nature of their role in society. The view of one group was that 'we are here to make society secure because these people are dangerously ill'. The other, slightly larger group, were less concerned about socio/political/administrative difficulties emphasising instead a more individualised therapeutic role which had at its centre the experiences of their patients. Management, of these two groups, espoused a rhetoric which favoured the latter but acted always in support of the former. As Steve Wright puts it:

> The perceived wisdom is that in order to secure the nurses' corner you have got to meet the management agenda. But the danger is that you become corrupted by the business ethos in the process and lose sight of what nursing stands for.
>
> (in Cole 1997: 26)

What it stands for is the key question and in the case of the two groups of forensic nurses, both were vociferous in their opposition to the *idea* of each other. Of course, neither group is right; neither is wrong. Everything would be easy if this were not the case. The problem is that there may be no such 'thing' as nursing, no locus of unity for its kaleidoscopic tasks, no defining characteristic at the heart of so noble an undertaking.

2 The whole truth?

The first thing that strikes you about task versus individual nursing debates is the individualist's contention that nursing operates within a holistic framework. According to this view, holism promotes an individual approach to care as well as identifying nursing as a caring profession. Nowadays few nursing texts fail to address the nature of care outside a holistic framework (see Jolley and Brykcznska 1992; Basford and Slevin 1995) and such frameworks have exerted a significant influence on the development of nurse educational criteria (Macleod Clark *et al.* 1996).

'Unarguably', say Davies and Lynch (1995: 394), 'there is a common nursing value that focuses on the wholeness of human beings.' According to Chinn (1987), 'the holistic view is now a central ideology of nursing' and, state Reed and Ground (1997), holism forms the basis of most current thinking in nursing.

However nurses seldom spell out the implications of their terms (Kitson 1988) and this can lead to unexpected conclusions. For instance does the term 'caring professions' presuppose health practitioners who are not caring? Or how is a caring profession different from the mass of ordinary people, for example relatives, who also care? Is there a sense in which the supposed uniqueness of one-to-one nursing relationships is an idealised construct? Could the hospital ward construed as a treatment centre also provide interventions which diminish pain and distress? Might not the technical efficiency of its staff or their dedication to hygiene, enhance feelings of safety and comfort? Conversely might not emphasising the individual encourage self-absorption or narcissistic distress?

The claim to holism

Primarily however, whatever the problematic nature of the phrase caring professions, it is the claim to holistic practice which makes a nursing ethics and therefore a nursing profession, however plausible, at least possible. It is the claim to holism which extends nurses' interests beyond medical technology and traditional concepts of patients as biological entities. No other professional group currently embraces holism as an adjunct to its putative status in society. Whatever the difficulties involved in discussing nursing as a caring profession, holism is the linchpin of its claim to autonomy from medicine. Undermine holism as a philosophical position and the central assumptions of some contemporary nursing groups collapse. Before addressing the philosophical issues however it may help to outline the basic tenets of holism and say something of its development within western thought. The problem with this is 'the difficulty of finding a clear statement of the central ideas of holism in the literature' (Phillips 1977: 2). There is also the corresponding difficulty of evaluating these ideas and making sense out of them. As Patterson (1998: 288) wryly observed, 'there is no succinct definition of holism, other than concepts which string together physical, spiritual, psychological and social needs and with an expression of emphasis on the interconnectedness of it all.' So what is holism?

The word itself stems from the Greek *holos* and means whole or complete, the 'w' being a late fourteenth-century addition (Pietroni 1977). Holism is the thesis that some wholes are more than the sum of their parts and that nothing true may be said about an organism unless it refers to that organism's whole. Any part which is cut off or set apart from the whole loses meaning.

The concept was introduced into western philosophy by Smuts in an attempt to show that matter, life and mind, 'so far from being discontinuous and disparate, will appear as a more or less connected progressive series of the same great process' (1926: 21). This process begins with evolution considered not only biologically but extending to the universe as a whole. According to Smuts, evolution nurtured an inner spirituality which determined its 'blossoming out' into greater wholes of which the universe, presumably, becomes its final parameter. Science, were it not so committed to analysis, said Smuts, would have acknowledged the point long ago.

Merely twenty years after the publication of Smuts' book, however, Bertrand Russell (1946) was condemning holism as the enemy of analysis. Russell objected to the notion that 'in order to know John, I must know all there is to know about John' since such a process of knowing could logically extend from John to the universe and no one can know the universe. If on the other hand one allows that there is only so much that can be known about John, then in a nursing context it makes sense to start with John as a patient since this makes sense of how a nurse might interact with him. Not to do this is to attribute importance to all aspects of John's life whilst neglecting what would ordinarily be important in a nursing context. To interact with John in such an unlimited way would make the appellation 'nursing' as we have known it in history difficult to apply. Further, operating within an unlimited perspective would cause pathology to lose its pivotal place. Historically pathology has dominated treatment settings and has profoundly influenced the ways in which nurses define their role.

Since the social contexts within which we evaluate the meaning of things is important, clearly nursing will be interpreted differently in medical circles as compared with for example educational or philosophical contexts. When called upon to apply nursing in medical settings, considerations of pathology take precedence because otherwise the entire hospitalisation and treatment endeavour collapses. That these treatments might be delivered in a cold, clinical and detached manner might constitute a failure of care – the hospitalisation and its treatment might be less pleasant for the patient – but this would not constitute a failure in the critical part of treatment which is to save life or cure disease and of course these interventions occur at the level of the patient's organs or bio-systems.

Also whilst many nurses are clearly concerned about holistic care, in practice their concept of it may be poorly worked out or, in medical settings at least, lip service alone may be all that is paid to it. Hermione Elliott (1997), Director of the UK Nurses Holistic Association, states that whilst holism is in the nursing curricula this may mean very little for although 'the words may be right' they occur in the absence of a true understanding of holism. Recognising this failure to realise the wider meanings of holism Barker (1995) pointed to the possible influences on holism embodied within eastern thought. He seemed to imply that nurses misunderstood holism's philosophical roots and that they had perhaps failed to consider it as anything more than another model or nursing process. This criticism is especially true of general nurses who, strangely eager to separate themselves from medicine, employ holism in an attempt to transcend the body when considering patient's needs. Conversely, psychiatric nurses have not displayed as strong an affinity with holism since they might justifiably claim to have already endorsed multi-dimensional approaches to care as well as having long ago extended their interests beyond the body. It is in this muddled context that we need to examine the antecedents of holism since the general effect seems to be one of obfuscation and uncertainty.

Having and being

Visiting Oxford in 1981 the literary critic Kenneth Tynan met the philosopher A.J. Ayer and suggested to him that western philosophies might learn something from their eastern counterparts. With 'Hegelian vehemence' Ayer dismissed eastern philosophies 'as having a minor, psychological interest only' thus endorsing the dominant western philosophical view. In his seminal text *Holism and Evolution* (1926), Smuts had barely mentioned the East even if his reasoning did occasionally resemble the transcendental qualities of eastern thought. For example his use of plants to illustrate important points is redolent of later holistic/humanist writing:

> we notice [in the plant] a unity of parts which is so close and intense as to be more than the sum of its parts; which not only gives a particular conformation or structure to the parts, but so relates and determines them in their synthesis that their functions are altered; the synthesis

affects and determines the parts, so that they function towards the whole; the whole is in the parts and the parts are in the whole.

(Smuts 1926: 86)

An approach which utilises all of the senses by definition contemplates the flower holistically. Not only does it understand the flower's evolution but it also experiences its smell. Holistically one communes with nature uncritically in the sense of not doing anything with it or to it. Quite simply, one is at one with it and with one's feelings and so on. Engler (1983) puts it this way:

> Instead of concentrating on one particular object, the meditator notes in a non-judgemental way each perception, thought, or sensation which enters awareness, observing the arising and passing of each mental object rather than the content of the object per se. Each perception, thought or sensation is simply observed without elaborating, commenting, judging, censoring, or giving it greater importance, based on its content, than any other mental event.

(in Hale 1997: 41)

In *To Have or to Be?* (1978), Erich Fromm also uses the flower to contrast eastern wholeness with the western commitment to analysis, reduction and ownership of knowledge. With the latter, the flower is broken down to constituent, functional, parts and understood in those terms, its environment (water, air and soil) similarly appraised in terms of functions and parts (the role of chlorophyll in the process of photosynthesis for example).

This cataloguing of knowledge is not just a question of westerners not being able to see the wood from the trees. Rather it is a consequence of post-Enlightenment thought whereby scientists have sought to explain data by identifying and labelling it as a prelude to manipulating and controlling it in the search for cause–effect relationships. Successive stages of this process require a reduction from one level down to the next so that explanations of human existence become ever more focused and tighter.

The case of schizophrenia

Scientists have attempted to explicate schizophrenia at the level of individual nervous systems or bio-chemistry in their search for a cure for the condition. Perceived abnormalities such as enlarged brain ventricles would be seen as having a causal effect on behaviour (Liddle 1994) which in turn would lead to the administration of drugs with the aim of promoting improved behaviour. The idea is not to disallow social or psychological factors completely but to stress their dependence on lower levels of explanation. Physiological advocates say that if we place our faith in science it will repay us with progress. Others point to the historical misuses of science, the intemperate leucotomies of the 1950s perhaps, the overdosing of patients with insulin or the more recent dialysis of schizophrenic patients' blood in the apparent belief that this would cleanse them of impurities. Contemporary psychiatric practices have similarly been criticised. User groups for instance have condemned diagnostic processes as well as what they see as an over-reliance on physical treatments.

Of course, non-medical explanations for schizophrenia have also figured in the history of psychiatry. In their different ways both Thomas Szasz (1974) and R.D. Laing (1965) have tackled conventional psychiatry's failure to attend to the experiences of patients and their political rights. However neither of these critiques provided much in the way of practical solutions to the behavioural and social problems which schizophrenia brings and whilst it is hardly the role of philosophical analysis to do this, one might have expected some nursing support for Laing's contention about the status of patients as persons. The reality is that the majority of psychiatric nurses remained faithful to a reductionist (biological) view of schizophrenia. This was a pity because here was an instance where a more holistic approach to patients might have been feasible. It would have required nurses to regard the explanatory power of medicine as *relative* however, to recognise that schizophrenia encompassed more than defective genes or brain abnormalities, to accept that any satisfactory approach to its treatment would be multi-disciplinary as well as based upon the patient's perceptions and needs.

Informal inquiry

A scientific approach alternatively examines the way in which *some* parts of an organism or entity can effect either itself or things outside itself. For example it will confidently assert the primacy of physical signs over and above whatever symptoms a patient may volunteer. Such analytic inquiries have their informal counterparts in how we solve our daily problems. Generally we achieve knowledge by applying, however haphazardly, rational principles to our experiences and in this way we are able to apply categories to what we observe, for example we objectify our perceptions such that we see a hard pillow or a red dress rather than redness or hardness per se. In general we appear intuitively receptive to notions of causality and relationships occurring over time and through space and we make our perceptions in the light of this. This preoccupation with causality however can lead to a neglect of other kinds of questions. Notice for instance how people see the question as eccentric if asked, 'Does a room continue to exist if nobody is in it?' Or, 'Does a tree falling in a forest make a noise if no one can hear it?' These questions provoke scepticism because they operate outside the laws of causation and measured relationships, deviating instead towards an infinite digression. The problem is that leaving empiricism (in its sense of verification) for matters not directly observable means entering a metaphysical realm whereby we become moral, inconclusive and evidence-less in our thinking, a realm in which the attribution of equal status to subjective and objective events becomes plausible, where discussions about the subjectivity of science are taken as valid.

Such questions acquired everlasting vigour following the crisis of doubt which began with the unleashing of Heisenberg's 'uncertainty principle' in 1927. Although Heisenberg's work cast doubt on a particular phenomenon in sub-molecular physics, the idea of a non-immutable world was sown, an idea which would grow into the pseudo-concept of multiple realities and a definition of science as just one of several ways to examine the world. A belief in multiple realities can be quite useful when opposing extreme scientistic exclusivity. However attempts to supplant *medical* science with alternative concepts drawn from humanistic philosophy still leaves the problem, as it did with Laing and Szasz, of the usefulness of these concepts in respect of specific medical ills. Most applications of scientific methodology continue to be firmly embedded in the Newtonian province of cause and effect and whilst uncertainty principles may be of interest to theoretical physicists, they play little part in scientific research. The same can be said for humanistic theories. Yet some nurses persist in abusing Heisenberg's formulation:

> There remains throughout the underlying belief of Heisenberg's uncertainty principle, that by observing an object, person or phenomenon we actually change it, which implies that we perhaps need to rethink our attitude towards, and the value we attach to, research within health and all caring professions.
>
> (Patterson 1998: 287)

One commonly encounters these attempts to dislodge the power of what is called the medical model and replace it with a more disseminated knowledge base. However, the extrapolation involved in these statements, from sub-molecular particles to health care systems, is not just implausible, it is breathtaking.

Theory and practice

Ethically, one would assume that within health care systems some consideration would be given to the manner by which ideas are likely to have an effect on practice. Critics of holism would point to its inability to ameliorate medical problems. An holistic approach might enhance the effects of treatment but in such cases it would simply be a euphemism for compassion, warmth, common sense and so forth. The point being that whereas eastern philosophies avoid a split between the subjective and objective, applying this principle to practical matters would simply turn the clock back. The fact is, that within transcendental frameworks the successes of modern medicine would not have occurred.

This is not to say that there exists a necessary relationship between theory and practice (Farrell 1981). For example whilst theoretically robust, psycho-analysis is of little practical use to many patients (Malan 1979). Behaviourism alternatively is quite useful at times albeit theoretically doubtful. Because carers are ethically obliged to respond to patients in ways which may be helpful they may therefore attach disproportionate weight to practical effects more so than to theoretical correctness. Or they may come to be suspicious of attempts to marry nursing to any one perspective.

In particular, efforts to restrict nursing inquiry to scientific, quantitative, approaches may lead to an avoidance of nursing interventions which appear to lack empirical validity but which may be valuable for other reasons.

Scruton (1995) observes that philosophers are obliged to ask questions which take human inquiry beyond evidence-based considerations. That is, whilst science may explain the antecedent or casual factors which precede events, questions may still be asked about the scientific process itself such as what constitutes a process or what is meant by an event. A philosophy of science examines the nature of the scientific process; it is not bound by that process. In his celebrated Reith Lectures Ian Kennedy (1981) applied moral reasoning to many of the assumptions and practices of contemporary medicine and his conclusions raised many doubts. Kennedy's critique could equally apply to nursing to the extent that nursing identifies itself with medical practice. Whether the critique could be applied as effectively to a nursing practice based on holism is debatable however. If nurses embrace a version of holism which is faithful to the fuller implications of its meaning, then this would relocate nursing away from medical concerns to a position where patients' experiences would be respected on their terms. It is the recognition of what this fuller holistic concept might ultimately entail which leads nurses to restrict their definitions of holism to multi-faceted or broad-based approaches to care, approaches which reflect a desire for multi-professionalism in an area of nursing historically dominated by medics. There may even be a sense in which adult nurses have internalised holism as a compact 'extra' whereby, in the fashion of giving a bed-bath, it becomes merely another element in the routine of nursing. In other words, 'that's the temperatures done', 'the medicines dispensed' and 'the holism apportioned'.

The main question

The main question is whether holistic nursing practice can be taken as grounds for consideration of nursing as a profession. That the nursing profession cannot have medicine as its knowledge base is obvious; another group already have that. That its knowledge base ought to be grounded in empirical data has been advocated by Gournay (1995). This however impedes the search for a nursing philosophy which has a concept of persons at its centre. The problem for practical nursing is that whilst holism provides a framework for multidisciplinary care based upon such a concept it hardly justifies assertions about a new nursing profession. Were this the case, then holistic prescriptions would stand some chance of implementation within medical settings. However, I suspect that nursing activities, be they holistic or not, are pursued in a context of there being no medical contraindication. Theoretically, holism *has* effected a measure of influence within nursing. However, as one encroaches upon areas of medical treatment the less influential it must be other than as a broader way of discussing what has already been decided medically.

Why challenge?

We could well ask why holism should challenge anything. By definition it complements medicine, absorbing its features into a wider consideration of patients' problems. However this overlooks the manner by which holism serves the interests of competing power groups. For example, holism challenges medical practitioners' historical first amongst equals position in respect of treating human ills. We may illustrate this by looking at the psychiatric disorder schizophrenia. Whilst not denying some relevance to social and psychological factors, on balance psychiatry allots the nervous system a primary, causative role in this condition. Holism alternatively posits a multiple causation and treats contributory factors with equal relevance. This being the case, one would expect holism to provide treatment approaches which reflect its position. However this is precisely the sort of practical requirement which has proved to be a stumbling block. As the *Annual International Medical Review* (1976) bluntly stated: 'The inability of physicians, psychiatrists included, to practice a genuinely holistic medicine that integrates knowledge of the body, the mind, and the environment is striking.' Whilst psychiatric nurses have, for well on thirty years, embraced a broad perspective to care the medical perspective, including within psychiatry, remains as dominant as ever. One curious explanation for this, according to Baruch and Treacher (1978) is that psychiatrists practise their own brand of 'holism' where they successively counter new or disparate ideas by a process of assimilation, a kind of disarming 'me too' response which has the effect of benevolently tolerating innovations whilst they either burn themselves out or are dissipated into ancillary professions such as counselling.

Holism and ethics

A contention of this chapter is that nurses clutch at holism because it is this which makes a nursing ethics viable and ethical codes are a basic ingredient of claims to professional status. However, if holism means that all have equitable value within a community, then how can nursing ethics be different from general ethics? For example, given that nursing is something which is

done by the population at large, there is a need to define professional practice separately from lay nursing. But how to do this given that nursing is an
activity which violently resists definition? Is it for instance the possession of
skills which differentiates these groups? Hardly, since it is undoubtedly true
that considerable skill attends much of what counts as lay nursing and in
any case claims to holistic practice rest on a denial of the primacy of medically
skilled interventions with patients. Further, we might inquire how skilled
interventions relate to general, for instance ethical considerations of care.

Specifically, if nursing skills were comprised of medical/surgical interventions, would caring for individuals require more than the implementation of
these skills? If technical skills were rehearsed in line with the latest developments, let's say in urology, would not the impetus to perfect such skills result
from the desire to care? Further, might not the efficient treatment of a
patient's organs or systems be synonymous with care? Even if delivered with
monotonous efficiency, does not the effort to acquire and maintain good
treatment skills equate with care? Indeed is not technical competence superior to that care which fails to avail itself of such skills? Putting this another
way, could not 'de-skilled' care be inefficient or even harmful?

Because nurses make close connections between holism and caring, it is
important to state that caring does not necessarily rest on holism; logically it
can't and indeed shouldn't. For if the point of holism is to care for the
person as a whole then what price the carer who lacks the technical capacity
to deal with what *ails* the person? And if the carer *can* deal with what ails
the person, is it necessary that they also care in that emotive sense with
which the word caring is typically loaded? It might be a bonus: it would
hardly be sufficient.

Kant (1949) had written that 'a good will is good not because of what it
performs or effects, not by its aptness for the attainment of some proposed
acts, but simply by virtue of its volition, that is, that it is good in itself'. In
other words, to witness someone do good unintentionally is of little use in
trying to estimate his or her virtue; intention is everything. But as Phillipa
Foot (1967) points out, a person's intention may hardly be the issue. Foot
holds that 'the disposition of the heart is a part of virtue' by which she
means that it is right to attribute moral failing to those who state, apparently
truthfully, that they *mean* to be helpful whilst being unable to be. It follows
that greater emphasis ought to be given to judging people's virtue as a function of their desires as much as their intentions and that therefore the will, in
this instance to care, must be understood in the sense of what is wished for
as well as for what is sought. Good intentions – to care, to be with, to
respect – are not enough. There must also exist a desire to be capable of
helping.

What I am saying is that words like 'holistic' edge aside medical pathology
as the defining characteristic of sick persons and that this would be fine if
the nurse could then utilise that holism so as to help the person overcome
the debilitative effects of their pathology. With holism however, the patient's

body is moved out of the focus of nursing with a consequent devaluation of the practical aspects of care (Bjork 1995). Attending to the non-physical aspects of patients' lives allows nurses to redefine these as important elements in the patient's condition. They may state for example that marital status or the work environment are central to understanding the patient's condition. The disease itself, be it physical or mental, is demoted. Being difficult to obliterate however, it is verbally, tortuously, stretched so that a stroke, for instance, is categorised as 'a transient but serious impediment to the upper circulatory system'.

Recently, a patient on traction was told that he was not ill: rather, he had 'a temporary and involuntary immobility contingent on environmental assault' (by a lorry). Similarly a student, during a placement in a hospice, was told in respect of an emphasis on health, that 'death was not an option'.

What these emphases do is abolish the patient's impediment as a human condition (Williams 1978) substituting instead a language of care which operates independently of that condition. Consequently there occurs a failure to attend to patients' sufferings as something incarnate in their pathology. Instead there emerge formulaic responses derived from a glut of nursing models and whose success depends upon considerations over and above patients' needs.

Students are quick to notice disparities between the needs of patients in treatment settings and the kinds of disembodied philosophies underpinning their training curricula. Charlotte Allen (1990: 43), for example, states that: 'Such [is] the focus on self and society, environmental health and sociolo-gese, that sometimes I have had to remind myself that we are not budding social scientists and that one day we will be nursing.'

Current emphases on quick treatment and discharge of patients also militates against holism and other person-centred approaches since these are time-consuming and difficult to measure. New developments in medical technology also reinforce medical dominance as well as multiplying the number of medical options available in respect of treatment. Medical practice is also distilled through specialisation and, from a holistic perspective, it becomes difficult to reconcile expertise organised around biological and anatomical systems with holism.

Prescriptive

The fact is, almost all nursing texts are prescriptive by nature (Johnson 1996) and nurses may not be doing what they say they are doing (Cormack 1983). Definitions of nursing competence typically stem from conceptual speculation and rarely from practice. Indeed, almost all nursing theories have evolved in relative isolation from observation or analyses of what nurses actually do. Barker's request that nurses examine the roots of holism is apposite but, on reflection, possibly misplaced given the propensity which nurses have for theories and models based upon individualised approaches to care. In general, nursing definitions of holism remain locked into the idea of individual patients considered from a variety of angles and, as suggested, with the medical angle retaining priority in treatment settings. Whereas, in respect of an eastern concept of holism, Yasmin Choudry (in Gorman 1995: 19) says that:

> The Asian concept is that we work in an holistic and spiritual way – you have the right balance of mind and body. The Western emphasis is on self, 'I', whereas the Eastern approach is on integration, 'we'.

It is unclear if nursing concerns are about a body–mind perspective or if current nursing usage represents, as I think it does, a pragmatic willingness to consider patients from different vantage points but with an ongoing emphasis on the patient's physical condition. It becomes hard to see whether *this* holism represents a genuine shift for nurses or is simply a fashionable acquiescence to academically driven rhetoric.

As Seedhouse and Cribb (1989) point out, interpretations of holism which emphasise alliterative or unorthodox approaches are not exclusive and many who call themselves holistic seem to happily function within conventional regimes. Graham (1990: 90) quotes LeShan who says that

> there is no such thing as an holistic technique or modality, only an holistic attitude – a concern to promote an understanding that all levels of a person's being: physical, psychological, spiritual, emotional, social and ecological are of equal importance in the prevention of disease and the quest for health, and that the potential for promoting health and overcoming illness resides within the person.

Most practitioners probably retain some allegiance to conventional medical regimes and might be reluctant to embrace philosophies in which the role of the self in illness is unduly prioritised. Indeed, preoccupation with the self has led to assumptions that certain illnesses are the result of living an 'unclean' life, eating meat, smoking and sexual excess. There is a resemblance here with primitive, mediaeval notions of possession and unclean spirits and the absence of objective rationales for dealing with people's ills. We live in an age of intolerance to the extent that some of us appear very willing to attribute responsibility to persons for their illnesses. Owen and Holmes (1993) observe that some holistic practitioners view the individual as someone who chooses experiences which will enhance his/her health. As such, collective forces which impinge on health are played down and it becomes the person's fault if they become ill. Indeed, Blattner (1981) goes further, saying that it is for individuals to choose whether they *want* illness or health. As Owen and Holmes note, this thinking implicitly endorses government policies and their cost-effective elements. Such thinking may even induce guilt in sick individuals who fail to recover from their illnesses.

Spiritual domains

As we observed, Ayer's objection to eastern philosophies derived from the unacceptability of uniting sense perception and cognition, a separation ingrained in western philosophy and psychology. Whilst the Buddhist unity of thinking and sensory experience violates no particular principle, its feasibility as a transcendent mechanism that enhances spirituality is basically a religious dimension. Of course the idea of spirituality is endemic within nursing. One thinks of care of the dying for example. It is compassion which motivates nurses to attend to the needs, including spiritual needs, of such patients.

If one embraces these factors (compassion, skill and vigilance) in one's approach to care then this might be called holistic. But it would be a 'closed holism', which is to say a holism which sets limits on what can be known about the patient whilst still extending nursing involvement. Closed holism does not imply any shift in how illness is conceptualised even when it requires nurses to act on their patient's behalf in ways not traditionally associated with nursing. Even so, some nurses might ponder the problematic nature of involving themselves with issues such as housing, unemployment, poverty and such like. Yet most nurses probably employ a closed holism since it permits a wider consideration of patient's problems. The nurse can, for instance, insist that a post hip-replacement patient not be discharged until relevant adjustments have been made to the patient's home. Or a psychiatric nurse could enable a patient to confront socio-economic problems seen as an obstacle to improvement. This kind of holism is summarised by Elliott (1997: 81–2):

> Holistic nursing recognises that health proceeds from a balance of our physical, spiritual, psychological and social needs. Our wholeness is dependant upon our relationship to each other, our environment and that which gives our lives meaning. Holistic nursing begins with an open mind and a willingness to explore the potential for personal growth and well-being for ourselves and others.

A holistic approach which would go beyond this would be one which questions the way in which illness is conceptualised. The problem with this 'holism proper' is that efforts to utilise it in treatment settings will conflict with medicine. For although medicine does not rule out alternative conceptualisations of human ills, even if radically different, it does reject any reduction in its authoritative capacity to diagnose and treat pathological conditions. Thus, whilst scientific medicine can be delivered in a warm and caring way, whilst it may take account of the views of multi-disciplinary teams, it can never be on easy terms with holism proper.

Other people's sources

Sokal and Bricmont (1998) have shown how some of the most influential thinkers of recent years have erroneously used theorems from the physical sciences so as to booster the face validity of their work. In nurse writing the trend seems to be to draw on principles which have their basis in spirituality or humanistic thinking. In both cases there is a patent refusal to explain why these terms are being used or to argue their relevance in respect of practice or even theoretical validity. Witness the following excerpt from Buckle:

> I believe it is possible to call orthodox nursing holistic, if this principle of caring for that spiritual part of us is incorporated into our nursing. Being spiritual does not mean being saintly, vegetarian, teetotal or believing in dogma. It simply means being whole.
>
> (in Schober 1995: 102)

Matters are somewhat more complicated with Kikuchi and Simmons (1996: 9):

> Making progress in nursing knowledge development plainly and simply depends upon nurse inquirers acknowledging that truth is all of a piece one indisputable whole that does not admit of contraries or contradictions.

Rew delves even deeper:

> Mercury [the metallic liquid] symbolises, for me, the unity of life that I believe is a truth in nursing. The individual drops, in constant interaction with each other, at one moment appear separate and autonomous. In the next, they collide and collude, forming communities that appear to act as a whole, then separate, once again, into dozens of singular bodies scampering across a seemingly thoughtless and impenetrable surface.
>
> (1996: 66)

According to Cloutier Laffrey (1996: 69) the 'interconnectedness of life is described as contiguous energy fields constantly interacting with one another and where no boundary is believed to operate between individual and their environments'. This meshing of language partly drawn from physics into discussions about social living is typical of humanistic nursing philosophy. The problem is that it is never made clear if we are dealing with metaphor, never made clear *how* energy fields affect social systems, never made clear what an impenetrable surface is.

The rhetoric of caring is also espoused with little regard for precision or meaning. Watson (1985) for instance sees the future of nursing as one where nurses aspire to a new consciousness of human caring, coming as a direct result of their challenge to the medical ideology. This tendency to identify scientific endeavour, in this case medicine but more usually physics, as an outcome of social construction and therefore just one amongst many myths is also endemic to a lot of nursing discourse. According to Watson, the 'human caring ideology' draws upon images of music and art and it has the aim of capturing metaphysical aspects of thought such as 'human centredness' and 'trans-personal caring'. Elliott accepts that 'when we get the relationship right everything else falls into place' and she links this with Neuman's (1989) philosophy of 'energy fields' and 'inter-linking and evolving authentic relationships'. She further quotes Watson:

> The nurse has a human responsibility to move beyond the patient's immediate specific needs and help the patient reach his or her highest level of growth, maturity and health. Nursing's most important goal is the promotion of self-actualisation.
>
> (Watson 1985)

Elliott (1997: 82) acknowledges that because these things can rarely be realised in practice, there occurs the concomitant temptation 'to dismiss them as lofty ideals, impossible to implement, with no relevance in the real world'. However she then counter-argues that nurses be trained in 'being' rather than 'doing' – thus the eastern influence again – and (drawing from Davidson-Rada and Davidson-Rada 1993) she suggests that nurses 'go beyond a focus on health or even well-being to one of infinite joy'. Now, I am not suggesting that such qualities be banished from nurse–patient relationships. Who would not want to be cushioned against unpleasant or difficult treatments by the provision of a civilised, compassionate, even spiritual environment? At the same time, one's attention is drawn to North's (1972) depiction of modern counsellors as 'the secular priests' and granted that healing is part of the nursing enterprise, it can hardly be what defines it as a profession – or can it? In what way, exactly, does the exercise of spiritual functions intrude on the traditional functions of nurses in treatment centres? How may joy be inculcated in students as part of their educational curricula? No one spells this out. That this preoccupation with quasi-mysticism, cosmic imagery and infinite joy is a natural outcome of holistic speculation is simply accepted.

It remains for holistic practitioners to tell us precisely *what* joy there is in being hospitalised? In being sick? Is there a sense in which suffering may be exalted? A sense in which the *experience* of being ill may be a condition where one's priority might not be to seek treatment but rather to seek to enter a 'new relationship' with illness through some inner understanding of what health means? As Schober (1995) observes, not everyone might want this, some might desire a cure for what ails them. Webb (1992) states that patients continue to value, and expect, good physical care and currently there is emerging, in mainstream journals, a dissatisfaction with what is seen as a neglect of basic nursing care (Harris 1995; *Sunday Telegraph* 1998). Morrison (1997: 5) comments that 'physical care is more important to patients whereas nurses argue for psycho-social care as being most important'.

No doubt nurses will continue to embrace holism as they continue to move away from their perceived dependence on medical doctors. They will persist in the belief that it is a viable philosophy by which to measure nursing interventions. However it is hardly that. For example it opposes common-sense notions of the world, it rejects analysis and it has not withstood the ordinary processes of philosophical inquiry very well. In any event it is a strange philosophy which resolutely struggles to explain the world of the nurse to the apparent neglect of the patient. If it forces a consideration of the patient as a human being, then this is fine albeit traditional concepts of decency and fair play would seem to be sufficient for that. That it might replace consideration of patients' religious needs with a dubious spirituality is regrettable. Finally, that it constitutes a new approach to medical ills and treatments is fanciful at best and at worst downright mischievous.

3 Carl's world

In 1992 I had the uncomfortable task of failing an unusually large number of students in their Registered Mental Nurse Final Examination. Whereas 10 to 15 per cent of candidates usually failed this examination, from the winter of 1992 about 40 to 50 per cent began to fail. Although students wrote well on their chosen topics and whilst syntax and grammar were generally fine, most of their responses were wildly inappropriate to the questions set. Whilst initially perplexing this development was eventually quite easily explained.

Bradshaw (1998) notes that ideologies which currently govern much of higher education are derived from the ideas of Illich (1975), Freire (1987) and especially the humanistic teaching of Carl Rogers (1980). Consistent with this, most questions on the nurses' examination paper had reflected Rogers' views on psychological counselling. In the winter of 1992 however, a fresh appointment was made to the question-setting panel and whilst this normally meant little change, on this occasion the questions dramatically altered in line with the new examiner's interest in psychoanalysis.

That many of the students had difficulty coping with the change was perhaps unsurprising. More surprising perhaps was the degree to which the thinking of British nursing students had come to depend on the ideas of an American counsellor–philosopher such that when examined from a psychoanalytic or cognitive science viewpoint, they continued to reproduce monologues to do with forming relationships, showing empathy, being non-judgemental and so on. It was not their fault. They had simply become the victims of that tendency in nurse education to accept new ideas as though the last word in truth (Robbins 1963) and in psychiatric nursing Rogers' views had, since the 1950s, achieved a quasi-religious status. More than anybody else it was he who had given counselling its language, contexts and ubiquity.

Critique

In order to evaluate Rogerian theory we must turn directly to Rogers himself. Of major importance is his fundamentalist Protestant upbringing because in many ways his later psychology amounts to a denial of this kind of Christianity with its stress on original sin and with man as a fallen, even predestined to fall, character. Indeed Rogerianism can be seen as a rejection of Protestant (Calvinist) predestination whilst putting in its place a version of Christianity with the judgement bits left out. Rogers' view of people is that they are constructed in such a way as to always choose to live in the world in ways which will be good. This is a central tenet of his philosophy, that persons will strive towards growth and fulfilment or what Maslow (1987) called self-actualisation. However, people could become blocked in their drive towards actualisation, events or feelings could conspire against them moving forward. Rogers saw the counsellor's task as intervening in these blocked states so as to help people 'get more in touch with their feelings'. In this way they could know better how to move on. How he went about this resulted in the biggest shake-up that psychotherapy has seen either before or since.

From psychotherapy to counselling

Rogers began by putting aside all notions of an objective reality either in terms of social rules or theoretical systems in favour of trying to understand people's subjective awareness of themselves and their place in the world. According to Thorne (1992), the trusting of his own experience had led Rogers to conclude that the experience of 'the other' merited equal trust and profound respect. Above all, he came to value personal experience: his own of course, but also the experience of others. There could be no higher calling than to develop an awareness of someone else's view of reality. From the beginning Rogers appeared unconcerned that this might entail having to respect *what* a person might be experiencing. Instead he concluded that theories which undermined processes of respecting others' awareness were anathema.

The attentive reader will spot the potential for conflict between Rogers' thinking as opposed to therapies which employ a knowledge base with attendant techniques or skills. Rogers disliked therapies which took this line arguing that one could only bring about change or growth in people by entering their experience. Eventually he came to believe that the *client* knows best which direction to take and that a significant aspect of the counsellor's role is to listen. The quality of that listening, of being with clients, would best be influenced not by erudition or technique but through a group of 'core conditions', namely empathy, acceptance and genuineness. These conditions would be the catalyst for the promotion of change in clients. Their introduction represented an important step in the development of psychotherapy and this is represented in the following two lists.

Psychotherapy
Knowledge
Academic qualifications

Professional language
Gravitas
Exclusivity
Technique

Counselling conditions
Genuineness
Empathy
Acceptance

At face value, the differences between these lists is stunning. Before Rogers, therapy was an intellectual, élitist and knowledge-based activity. There now emerged a veritable playground of emotions, therapeutic engagements that are as much about feeling as reasoning. The essence of this view is that if one has an experience which one can trust, then one simply trusts it and by so doing 'one validates experience as a basis for actions which flow from it'. Hence, a series of conditions emerge which appear to have little to do with education, learning, structure and so on. This being the case we may ask if this means abandoning training as a prerequisite to practising counselling or, as Shanley (1988) puts it, whether there might exist 'inherently helpful people' who have little need of preparatory training. As it turned out training courses in counselling burgeoned to the point where these days they are as freely available as courses in chiropody. Part and parcel of this popularisation of course was the shifting of the balance within therapeutic relationships so that, from a Rogerian perspective, they could now be seen as encounters within which both participants could be considered equal. This 'dethroning the therapist' is seen by many writers (Kirchenbaum 1979; Thorne 1992) as Rogers' most 'revolutionary' contribution.

Genuineness (or congruence)

Rogers believed that this condition was the most critical to the counselling enterprise (Thorne 1992). It means the absence of facade, a sense in which the counsellor's presence is transparent to the client insofar as the counsellor allows his thoughts, feelings and attitudes to flow freely within the relationship. It could be likened to a duet for one, with the client ultimately as chief beneficiary. Of course, it is acknowledged that the counsellor is in touch with his negative as well as his better feelings but in bringing these bad feelings into the open, he hopes that they too will melt down in the warmth of the evolving relationship.

This stance, whilst plainly at odds with the kinds of psychotherapy which went before has some roots in older existentialist therapies. However it is plainly a departure from psychoanalysis where the therapist is a kind of fountainhead of wisdom, power and so on. With Rogers, all of these elements are shared or owned by both client and counsellor. Such a concept of sharing can lead to misunderstanding. For example, what happens if the counsellor simply off-loads negative feelings on to the client? What if he (genuinely) blurts out that he hates the client? Apparently, this is not what being genuine means. What it actually means is that the counsellor gets in touch with his feelings in the sense that he does not deny to *awareness* those aspects of them which are uncomfortable. The level of awareness is important here. According to Nye (1992: 112) the communication processes between client and counsellor can operate at levels in which 'meanings just below the level of the client's awareness' come into play. To bring this about, says Nye, the counsellor must genuinely feel his way into the different core conditions such that any 'attempts to artificially manipulate conditions in the therapeutic relationship are not likely to be successful: the therapist has to be real'. The problem with this is how do you *be* genuine? Either you are genuine or you are not. It is not something which you can *be*. Further, could one feign an emotion or deliberately lie if one genuinely believed that this was the right thing to do? Also, what evidence is there that non-Rogerians hide behind their therapist role any more than Rogerians do? Could not the Rogerian stance of 'standing outside the therapist role' be as much a role as any other? As Goffman (1972) would put it, by what mechanisms are Rogerians freed from the constraints of the ritualised and dramatic requirements of 'the presented self'? Rogerians provide no account of how the counsellor comes to know his genuineness from his ulterior motives. All told, a concept of genuineness seems fraught with psychological difficulties.

Acceptance

This condition concerns what has been called 'unconditional positive regard', the process of accepting clients without preconditions. As Thorne (1992: 3) observes, it constitutes an acceptance which is 'totally uncontaminated by judgements or evaluations of the thoughts, feelings or *behaviour* of the client' (emphasis mine). Of course, most of us have probably never experienced this kind of acceptance. Intuitively it appears to be such a sweeping concept that its widespread application within human affairs seems unlikely.

Can one really have a regard for someone which is unconditional, which could be applied to anybody regardless of who or what they were? Even in the case of loved ones, the idea of *unconditional* acceptance must stand as psychologically implausible. Intimate relationships incur elements of rejection, cost benefit exchanges, blame, guilt and so forth. Indeed the more one thinks about Rogerian acceptance the more dubious it becomes.

This particular difficulty has not gone unnoticed by followers of Rogers. Thorne, for example, lists 'defensive, aggressive and vulnerable' clients as especially problematic to which one could add evasive, anxious, depressed, elated and so on. Note, however, the psychological nature of the problem categories selected by Thorne. Observe the manner by which reprehensible *behaviours* are left out. What to do for instance if one's client is a rapist? Or if the client is sexist or racist? How does one accept someone who has committed sexual acts against children and who tells you that they intend to do it again? What if a client is just plain nasty? Does the counselling regime still require that one accepts him or her unconditionally?

Almost certainly, counsellors would reject the notion of acceptance masquerading as forgiveness. However this raises the question that if the client is a rapist, then should he not be asking for forgiveness? Is it not morally questionable to provide him with a confessional forum in which it appears as if he is being forgiven albeit the language has been changed? My view is that counselling can be a moral undertaking inasmuch as it provides forms of absolution in those cases where some violation of the moral order has occurred.

According to Nye (1992) acceptance cannot extend as far as forgiveness because one does not evaluate all of a person's behaviours equally; one can reject some behaviours whilst accepting others or reject some behaviours whilst accepting the person overall. Nye gives the classic example of a parent who criticises a child's misbehaviour whilst continuing to love the child. Counsellors make great use of this principle of rejecting the behaviour whilst accepting the person. It constitutes for them the primary 'get out' clause for dealing with morally objectionable behaviours. However, the possession of good qualities does not necessarily mitigate the bad. Further, the idea that we might regard the transgressions of strangers in the same way as those of our children seems a weird idea at best. The point that is ignored is that it matters little that Hitler was a lover of art, animals or children, apparently true on all counts. What matters is that he was Hitler. Although the performance of good actions may mitigate the presence of bad, this can only occur where the bad actions have been adjudged to be outweighed by the good. The point being of course that they still deserve to be judged. There are at least some whose behaviours merit little acceptance, at least not without attaching conditions, and it is to Rogers that much of the responsibility must go for the kinds of permissiveness which now, as a society, we seem to be trying to put behind us.

Empathy

Phenomenology and existentialism are the philosophies which most closely resemble Rogerian thinking and which directly relate to the concept of empathy.

Phenomenology is about inquiry; existentialism is about choice. The nature of this inquiry is that it tries to reduce to essentials that which we wish to inquire about. We must search for the truest meaning of things by dispensing with those meanings which have come to us through learning. We must separate what is intrinsic to the mental state from what is external to it. Our consciousness is related to the world of course, but in the sense of what we intend in the world. Man's existence, as Husserl (1964) has it, is what he purports to be. Thus, he must choose.

Existentialism differs from phenomenology in that it sets itself the task of working out our existence without recourse to modernist theories or scientific approaches. It puts us in the awkward position of having to make choices, choices which have consequences for others as well as ourselves. As such, existentialism is about the problem of being in the world. As Hamlyn (1987: 323) observes of Heidegger:

> By stressing the idea of being in the world as a fundamental notion, it may seem that Heidegger is trying to abandon the Cartesian framework and to emphasise the necessity of accepting the idea of a common world as a precondition of all else.

That being the case, the property of what is true is always mine. Other people, their behaviours and statements, obtain credence only by how they are perceived by me.

In a very real sense, following Sartre, it can be said that one chooses one's world. The problem, as Sartre himself bitterly observed, is that 'Hell is other people', by which he meant that one must experience the torment of choosing in a world where others choose as well. This essentially philosophical problem is only marginally helped by Rogers placing it within psychological practice. In essence, what Rogers does is personalise age-old philosophical problems: Why am I? Who am I? Where am I going? How do I get there? Am I alone? And so on. The questions are real enough and have withstood analysis for hundreds of years. The problem is that their transformation into a counselling parlance by Rogers involved a neglect of the intellectual rigour which had customarily attended their inquiry and the substitution instead of a set of feeling states and a startling new terminology. Suddenly, age-old philosophical questions obtain credibility as functional elements within an 'organismic striving' for integration and wholeness – the word organismic was never explained by Rogers – and are worked out on an 'emotional field of experience'. There emerges a system which begins with unprovable assumptions, relinquishes responsibility for verifying these assumptions whilst substituting instead the risky proposition that true verification stems from experience. As Brewster Smith (1967) says, all that this leads to is personal description since phenomenology cannot explain events (nor does it seek to, of course). However hard we might try to look at our own consciousness objectively, it becomes difficult to see how we escape subjectivity, even momentarily, so as to do this. When we do reflect on consciousness what we invariably find is that it is directed towards some end. That is, we are never merely conscious but are instead conscious of some *thing*. We are perpetually trapped in the act of attaching meaning to the objects of our existence. So that when Rogers claims that 'the locus of psychological causation lies entirely within the phenomenal field of conscious experience' he is correct up to a point. What he overlooks is the extent to which we are socialised into making sense of our society in the way that we do. However we may note the intrinsic attractiveness of Rogers' position. After all, it accords with the fact that many people see psychology as something which focuses on personal experience as well as providing a basis by which people might aspire towards change. However in order to change we must first choose and it is this element which brings Rogers closer to existentialism in that if we choose *not* to choose, then we entail a loss of being in the world. Whereas by choosing, we make real in the world just exactly who we are, irrespective of the social forces which bear upon us. By refusing the responsibility of choice, however, we engage in what Sartre calls 'bad faith' or what Rogers – lacking Sartre's poetry – called a block to organismic growth. In the case of counselling it seems implicit that inasmuch as the client has chosen, he/she has chosen well.

If the idea of empathy is that the counsellor enters without misgivings the private world of the client, then in the case of nasty clients this is surely going to be difficult. Is empathy possible for example with someone who has committed rape? Might it be particularly awkward if the gender of the counsellor and the victim were the same? It seems that whatever empathy one brings to counselling will vary depending on the background (gender, sexual maturity, age) of those involved. Dalrymple's (1995) male patient who beat up his girlfriend 'because she was doing my head in' is a good example of self-determination in Rogerian terms. In this case the patient sought acceptance and empathy from his doctor on grounds of girlfriend-induced stress.

How does a counsellor not judge such behaviour? Perhaps the counsellor chooses not to judge but, if so, is not that a judgement also?

The problem with phenomenology

If the world was dependent on my view alone, then my view would constitute all men's views. There would be no need for counselling since all of us would be free (from distress) by virtue of choosing freedom. Logic entails that we would not choose either physical or psychological confinement. However, to choose freedom is to impinge on the freedom of others. Also, in making one's choice, one concedes the rightness of doing so and, therefore, the rightness of others to do so as well. However, in respect of others choosing freedom, a loss of one's own freedom as a result of their choice may occur. We may not seek to infringe other people's liberties but in furthering our ambitions we may do so nevertheless. For most of us, daily living is a process of (often painful) negotiation around those with whom we interact. Clients in counselling are not immune from this. They know that there are others outside the counselling relationship whose choices may disagree with their own. The counselling process therefore would seem to require a suspension of belief in the awkward compromises of the outside world. In effect, a kind of psychological reductionism operates to exclude the various social forces which might contradict the counselling process or its outcomes.

Woolly thinking

According to Joel Kovel (1978) the humanistic movement generally is defined by its lack of system. Kovel likens Rogers' therapy to 'an overarching mood', at heart a combination of old European existentialism and the American desire for the perfectibility of man. It is a process whereby latent powers are liberated so as to enable people to choose different directions in their lives. It is a means by which the ways of the world are transcended by a faith in the immutable spirit of man.

Although, at first sight, this seems innocuous enough with its built-in assumptions about inherent goodness, there is a sense in which Rogers becomes 'the new Nietzsche', trumpeting mankind's increasing mastery over destiny as he/she aspires ever onwards towards self-actualisation (Tanner 1994).

On the other hand, little attention is paid to what the consequences of counselling relationships might mean for those involved. According to Rogers (1951), 'the end of counselling is the process and the end is not to be sought anywhere but the process'. As Halmos (1965: 156–7) notes, here is one apostle for whom the pedestrian notion of separate means and ends does not exist. The means *are* the end and the end, what ever it may be, is justified from experience and not by social norms or constrictions.

Of course, what actually occurs in counselling may be more prosaic than this. There may well be attempts to deal with problems which directly refer to the world outside. However my criticism is that this outside world will reflect little more than the subjectivity of the individuals involved and that the real problem would be how to reconcile the subjectivity of the individual to wider social contexts.

In any event who is this 'individual'? It is not easy to see how anyone could embody the kind of flesh and blood individualism of which Rogers speaks, other than within the counselling conditions which he espouses. Because these conditions are artificially contrived, client improvements are likely to be short-term since re-entering the mainstream of life will involve confronting discrepancies between the individual's new perceptions or attitudes and the vicissitudes of ordinary life.

The task of human perception is to construct recognisable forms be they objects or persons. Making sense of these objects involves attributing properties to them such as 'this is a tree', 'this is a train' and so forth. Our perceptual processes depend on a range of factors both inherent (constancy factors) and social (personal interest and occupational). By utilising Heider's (1958) attribution theory we can also infer relationships between the properties we perceive. For instance, 'the falling tree crushed the car'. According to Heider, the sorts of mechanisms which underpin the attribution of causality are 'similarity', 'closeness' and 'consistency'. This means that to attribute a causal relationship between a person and an act, it would be necessary to observe that person across a range of social encounters. If we already knew that someone is good we could of course forego the need to witness their good behaviour in different settings. In Rogerian practice however, one finds a complete reversal of this. Instead one discovers the tendency to 'hold a good person responsible for good acts' even though both counsellor and client, being relative strangers, possess only their experience of each other in isolation.

Research

Perhaps Rogers' second important contribution to therapeutic practice was to expose his work to outside scrutiny, a practice which until then was unheard of in psychotherapeutic practice. In doing so it appears that he was attempting to place his work within empiricist traditions in research. This was a curious thing for him to do because it involved an implicit acceptance of the role of determinacy in psychotherapy. Although Rogers' views on this are complex (Nye 1992) and even confused (Kovel 1978) this is hardly surprising in someone who believed that determinism and freedom to choose are by no means opposites. Cohen (1997: 231) observes that Rogers could be quite pious about the reluctance of other branches of psychotherapy to test their theories, psychoanalysis famously so. This, in my view, is probably nearer the truth which is that it was one-upmanship which lay behind his apparent acceptance of the role of determinism and that there is little to suggest that he was truly committed to it. Probably he wanted the kudos which his research innovation would bring but without conceding his basic attachment to phenomenology.

As a therapist, Rogers had committed himself to the autonomous status of his clients and he would therefore have had to accommodate this belief with his new-found discovery of determinism. He did this by weighting determinism more heavily during the early stages of counselling. He had reckoned that to be maladjusted is to be less free to choose. On entering the counselling relationship however, the client begins to harmonise the self with what lies outside, begins to choose his way out of distortion becoming less defensive as the counselling proceeds. At the same time, the act of choosing is also determined in the sense that it is affected by prevailing conditions both prior to and accompanying the act of choosing. Thus the inevitability of a self-actualising choice which is something chosen but at the same time something which one *has* to choose.

Rogers' upbringing provides some clues as to how he came to these conclusions.

As a young man he had rejected the mid-western religion of his family with its stark principle of predestination, the Calvinist doctrine that one's salvation has been worked out already. At its simplest level this doctrine holds that God must know who is or is not saved. This is a dreadful thought, the notion that whatever one does, one may be doomed anyway. However, predestination has the powerful effect of forcing one to do good works because herein lies the psychological assurance of salvation, for in the midst of my good works and the avoidance of bad, how can I be anything *but* saved? The implications for Rogers' position are that in developing a system in which self-actualisation (a kind of earthly salvation) played such a large part, he was turning away from the dreadfulness of predestination with its morbid anxiety, its sense of loss, its apprehension of inevitable judgement. Instead, man is seen as always striving towards goodness, always choosing right from wrong. As Joel Kovel remarked, Rogers would appear to have cast out the devil from human affairs.

Evil

Rogers' detractors continuously taunted him with his reluctance to address the question of evil. Of course, he never answered this at all (Cohen 1997) preferring instead to press on with his beliefs about inherent goodness. Whilst frequently acknowledging that people could be vicious or destructive he recoiled from the notion of evil unredeemed. Man could and would transcend evil, it was in his nature to do so, to realise his better potential and actualise his positive self. Superficially this seems okay and you might begin to wonder what there is to object to. At a deeper level, however, it denies the place of rational thought in everyday life and especially how this might help us formulate a moral code by which to lead a reasonable social life.

A striking example of Rogers' distrust of reason occurred during an interchange with his son-in-law, Larry Fuchs. Once, when trying to say something meaningful to Rogers, the 'great listener' (Cohen 1997: 186–7) continued to thumb through a magazine. Cohen quotes Fuchs telling Rogers that: 'For a humanist to constantly deride reason, as I find you doing, in order to make your point that people hide their feelings and are therefore less human seems not only unnecessary but harmful.' Apparently, Rogers had accepted a comparison between concentration camps and American universities since it allowed the person making the comparison to rid himself of some anger.

Of the same generation as Rogers, Hugh Dudley (1996: 268) wrote:

> Many of us have had difficulty in understanding man's inhumanity to man. Yet my own experiences in the Far East in the late sixties have forced me to the view that it is the exception to find that the human race is good. There is a long and complex argument here on the matter of sin and redemption, but I believe that it is right to adopt the negative stance that man is bad though whether there is the possibility of perfection, only the slow if inexorable march of natural selection – perhaps modified by the feedback from humans themselves – will establish.

That is to say, questions of good and evil are things which we discuss and not in any great expectation that that discussion will lead to the abatement of evil. Since, for Rogers, there is no objective reality or, to put it another way, 'as many realities as there are persons' (Cohen 1997: 221) such discussions become redundant as indeed they must within a system which has no need of ethical or logical rules by which to guide our actions. With Rogers, one presumably trusts that one is right or, to use the jargon, one 'goes with the flow'.

Vietnam

There have been two biographies of Rogers to date and the Vietnam War does not figure in either of them although there is an oblique reference in Cohen (1997: 209). This is hardly surprising considering that this war represented the death of everything Rogers held dear. This was no European conflagration, no expression of an old world pessimism fuelling Freudian aggression and despair. These were Americans dropping napalm on rural communities in the name of 'making the world safe for democracy'. In so doing, did it not occur to him that people might pursue their own ends at the expense of others and that in so doing they would seek to justify their actions by pleading a higher good? If Rogers' teaching can be seen as a homespun (American) philosophy, a philosophy of becoming, of choosing a lifestyle – always positive, always life-enhancing – then how did he reconcile this with his country's involvement in Vietnam? Was he so sure that people can capably distinguish between that which is a higher good and base self-interest? As David Pilgrim says, 'It takes a steady eye to see that the extermination of native American Indians and the razing of Vietnamese villages were the opposite side of the same coin of a cultural commitment to the freedom of the individual' (1997: 81). To the extent that Rogers interested himself in political issues, he appears to have concentrated on world affairs, visiting different countries including the USSR (always an easy mark for western psychologists) and inviting Protestants and Catholics from Northern Ireland to America. Apparently he believed that what the Northern Ireland problem needed was about two hundred encounter groups. When Rogers did refer to Vietnam it was to inform Defence Secretary Robert McNamara (see Cohen 1997: 207) that he misunderstood the passion of a smaller enemy's beliefs largely because such passion is missing from the American educational system. We are, I presume, meant to believe that a secondary school curricula based on Rogerian principles might have influenced American military policy.

In mitigation, most Americans of his generation had no social or other collective disasters upon which to draw, neither the carnage of two world wars nor, like many of the European psychoanalysts, generations of anti-Semitism. This is not to say that American life lacked malevolent or tragic dimensions but whatever these might have been they appeared to pass Rogers by. It may be relevant that he was born and reared in the American

mid-west which is usually seen as the most socially and politically isolation-
ist part of America.

Accepting Rogers' ideas

Several factors made the acceptance of Rogers' ideas likely but none more so
than the way in which he watered down any need for a knowledge base. Here
was a therapy which did not require a lengthy training involving the uptake
of knowledge or a prolonged personal therapy. Previously, entry to therapist
training had been restricted so that those permitted to practice were small in
number. This is not to say that Rogerian training is feeble or patchy but that
given its disdain for theory, its devotion to feeling, it was inevitable that its
preparatory courses would quickly spread. That being the case, there are
probably now as many counsellors as there are double glazing salesmen and
with no shortage of people needing their help. It may be true that liberating
psychotherapy from the clutches of medicine and orthodox psychology was
a great service and one recalls at this point Freud's insistence that lay-
persons as well as just doctors could practice psychoanalysis. Stringent
requirements on Freudian practice subsequently emerged however and
American analysts still insist on its practitioners being medically qualified.
In fairness, recent years have seen attempts to register counsellors, count
heads and regulate courses.

The notion that anyone can do it still prevails however and, for example,
Britain's most popular nursing journal, *Nursing Times*, continues to adver-
tise counselling courses via correspondence.

Thorne (1992: 65) notes the vociferous reaction to what some saw as
Rogers, in effect, giving away their livelihood:

> Profound issues of power are at stake in these conflicts and the accusa-
> tions of superficiality or of irresponsibility are a scarcely veiled attempt
> to silence someone who calls into question the authority of psycholog-
> ical knowledge. The radical belief that it is the client who knows what
> hurts and how to find healing throws a mighty spanner in the works for
> those who see it as their task to evaluate 'conditions' and to set up
> programmes to remedy problems.

I doubt if Rogerianism even remotely influenced the practice of conventional psychiatry or psychology. What Rogerianism did do, perhaps, was
devise a way of no longer restricting psychotherapy to the sick. Recast in the
guise of counselling it was now something which could be directed at helping
people to become happier. Rogers must have known that the juxtaposition
of therapy and happiness made no sense, that 'therapeutics' implies some
intention to cure. As Thorne favourably observes however, to cure is to exercise
authority and this Rogers and his disciples rejected. To a large extent, Rogers'
reforms took place against a background of a vigorous counter-culture which

was anti-authoritarian in general. Alternative, radical changes to traditional power bases were constantly mooted and the hierarchical nature of psychiatric power was a favourite target. The germination of Rogers' ideas stretches back further than this of course. But it is in the cultural maelstrom of the 1960s and later that his ideas began to gel. Objections to conventional interpretations of authority intensified following President Kennedy's assassination and a paranoia/conspiracy ethos which took root in the lone assassin view favoured by establishment forces. Any therapy which deprived experts of their received wisdom could hardly fail to attract its share of devotees. Rogers suited the turbulence of his times and the easy accessibility of his counselling approach made him the most adored helper in history.

Critique

Thorne (1992) notes Buber's (1937) objection that Rogers is about inventing individuals rather than persons, that his is a religion without a God, a secular humanism in which men and women become their own Gods. In addition, he notes how Rogers courts danger by accepting his client's statements as true. Thorne (1992: 75) interprets this and other critiques as general attacks on psychotherapy – true but irrelevant – and he notes that Masson's (1990) criticisms are particularly cynical and extreme. It is hard to refute the charge of cynicism. However the charge of extremism is unfounded when you consider Rogers' response to criticisms being to point to, time and again, his experiences as a therapist. Indeed, his entire worldview seemed to stem from the 'logic' of his therapy sessions. He rarely stepped outside of this world although occasionally he did let slip a more ambivalent side to his nature.

> It disturbs me to be thought of as an optimist. My whole professional experience has been with the dark and often sordid side of life, and I know, better than most, the incredibly destructive behaviour of which man is capable. Yet that same professional experience has forced upon me the realisation that man, when you know him deeply, in his worst and most troubled states, is not evil or demonic.
>
> (Rogers 1958: 17, in Thorne 1992: 80)

I believe that this is true at many levels; levels of ambiguity, of doubt, of inability to choose and so forth. I accept that a capacity for good exists even in the presence of evil. However, whilst this late concession to ambiguity does not rule out the possibilities of evil, it still does not explain why it is *always* right to embrace the good side of a dual nature in the way that Rogers said was necessary. For Thorne (1992: 44) these objections are seen as perversity, a common enough reaction amongst counsellors. However, the issue is not one of rejecting the helpfulness of acceptance and empathy as basic reactions to people in trouble. Nor do I desire any letup in voluntary undertakings such as help for addiction groups, women's groups, AIDS and other illnesses, the Samaritans, Relate, bereavement and so on. Such organisations constantly prevail against human tragedies and to denounce them would be absurd. Rather is the issue about rejecting an unworldly idealism which has no room for evil or malevolence and where aggression and hatred persist because not confronted.

A lack of rigour

Rogers knew that others saw him as soft-headed, cultist, non-academic, non-rigorous, full of empty ideas about the self and wishy-washy notions of goodness. But, as both Thorne (1992) and Cohen (1997) make clear, whilst constantly reminded that the world's evils cast shadows over his discourses on goodness and love, he simply took no notice. In fact, he appeared to focus his anger at the idea that you had to be a doctor in order to practice psychotherapy, an objection which he shared with Freud. But this was a winnable argument. In general he avoided the more difficult philosophical issues which his teaching raised. In his wake, there proliferated books, papers and conferences all extolling the virtues of counselling to the extent that nurses especially came to see his views as not open to question.

Most counsellors whom I have met are entirely decent individuals even if, occasionally, a bit too sweet to be wholesome. There is nothing wrong in befriending people or even in charging money for it and it is a sad fact that for some, counselling will be their first opportunity to be listened to. If the client or patient *believes* that it does them good, fine. However, that kind of belief can leave you vulnerable to manipulation and exploitation, not the least of which is due to that immodesty which persuades some people that they are experts in human relationships. Such an expertise seems implausible to me and my feeling is that it works best as a kind of cushion for people whose proclivity is for 'feeling good about feeling bad'. Professor O'Hear (in Walden 1998: 9) captures well the dislocation of reason during the aftermath of the death of Princess Diana: 'Feeling was elevated above reason, caring above principle, personal gratification above commitment and propriety.' Naturally, some may see only good in this. They might perceive the ascendancy of counselling as denoting a more caring society. This is a superficial reading of its role however. A stricter interpretation would regard it as having been instrumental in bringing about relativism in social affairs as well as responsibility for the pernicious idea that actions can be justified from feelings alone.

4 Flowers in their mouths

... saying the words 'I care about you' isn't necessarily a reflection of the truth, although many disappointed lovers have learned this lesson the hard way.

(Adler *et al*. 1980: 81)

Breaking and entering

Most research is grounded in personal experience (Robinson 1987). Research which lacks a 'biography of the investigator' ultimately becomes 'so much hollow ritualist cant' (Lofland and Lofland 1984). It is biography which lends work its substance and integrity. Accordingly, I want to outline my involvement with a group of nurses claiming to implement a therapeutic community within a secure, forensic, unit. In particular I want to say how and why I gained entry to this community so as to examine what the nurses were doing and see whether it matched what they said they were doing.

A biographical note

Who can be sure about what attracts them to working with people who are mentally disturbed? I had always been fascinated by psychiatry, drawn towards notions of madness and its possible meanings. Whether this belies some desire to apprehend my own madness is something I'm not sure about. I do know that my involvement in psychiatric nursing was never entirely rational. Frank spoke about what had drawn him to psychology: 'a bit of fascination about the catastrophic effects of mental illness and what it can make people do'. A social worker, Donald, aptly expressed the kinds of feelings which underline these sentiments: 'Attitudes about dangerousness. There's an unacknowledged part of me which has them being mad for me so that I can use my job as a social boast.' Biggs, an occupational therapist, talked about: 'Deeply disturbed people – I link into parts of me – that's why I have the mood swings. Sometimes it's I'm not worthwhile, everything I do is valueless, worthless.'

Previous work

I had long cultivated an interest in the development of therapeutic communities in Britain and had written about the open door movement of the 1950s (Clarke 1993). So when a forensic unit called Ambrose pronounced itself a therapeutic community I decided to investigate the extent to which therapy, under locked conditions, might be feasible. These forensic units had been set up following the recommendations of the Butler Committee (1974, 1975). By the early 1970s many agencies had long recognised deficiencies in dealing with mentally abnormal offenders (Glancy 1974). Courts often had little choice but to imprison or consign such offenders to State Hospitals such as Broadmoor. Following Butler's recommendations, Regional Health Authorities were urged by the then Secretary of State, Barbara Castle, to construct conditions of security at local level for such patients and, reluctantly (Snowden 1983; Pilgrim and Eisenberg 1985) they complied. These units would vary in terms of size, staffing complement, architectural layout and security considerations although Fuller (1985) noted that Home Office Rules and Court Orders would apply to them uniformly. Additionally, Bluglass (1978) observed that units would be at the mercy of local demographic pressures, for example urban adjacency and the public's fear of violence. Yet the hope was to avoid 'mini-Broadmoors' by providing ample staff ratios. In general, proponents of these units saw them as bridging a yawning gap in psychiatric provision.

Although both Sharp (1975) and Grey (1973) had identified the therapeutic community as an influence on prison reform, Butler (1974, 1975) played down its suitability for the kinds of aggressor offenders who would inhabit the new units. Since the essence of therapeutic community practice typically involved management by group processes and a somewhat relaxed approach to relationships within organisations, Butler unsurprisingly opted for a rehabilitative regime designed to reorient patients towards good, adaptive, social behaviours. In general, neither Butler (1975) nor Glancy (1974) were able to provide guidelines as to the relative balance of therapy versus security. Butler had noted the general public's overriding concern with physical dangerousness but failed to define it. In particular, said Butler (1975: 74): 'A balance has to be struck between the need to protect society and the right of the individual to return to the community when his detention is no longer strictly justified.'

On the issue of dangerousness and the protection of society therefore, the way was left open for arguments about how the balance should be tilted and in which direction. In the absence of guidelines, the issue would be resolved haphazardly. A Charge Nurse stated:

There is no scientific way of demonstrating a level of dangerousness in an individual, no formula. ... Most decisions are based on feelings. If someone is making a parole decision there is no graduated process of evaluation. It's a question of feeling but the public should be satisfied.

May and Kelly (1982) have identified nurses' reluctance to accept forms of sociopathic behaviour as illness with a tendency towards punitive responses as occasions demand. Sociopathic behaviour, in effect, refuses to legitimise the therapeutic intentions of nurses and it was against this confused picture that Ambrose Unit had styled itself a therapeutic community of the 'Rapoport' or 'Henderson' type. According to Fuller (1985: 47) '… the official labelling of an establishment is [hardly] a reliable guide to what it comprises: organisational identity cannot be assumed but requires objective description and comparison'.

It was the veracity of this claim which fascinated me, the improbability of therapeutic community practice within a locked system of care. Other, less bookish, sources also fuelled my interest. For instance shortly before writing this, I overheard a discussion between two of the Ambrose nurses.

1st nurse: The patient will be okay if we can get her in and check her out ourselves.
2nd nurse: Yeah, provided we can keep 'you know who' well away from her.
1st nurse: (*sarcastically*) Our therapeutic community angels!
2nd nurse: (*menacingly*) Well you know what happens when that lot put their oar in.
1st nurse: You just can't believe it sometimes. Mitchell (*a detained patient*) was practically climbing the walls – he hit someone yesterday – and Miss Florence Nightingale (*a proponent of the therapeutic community*) wanted to talk to him: talk to him! How fucking stupid can you get?

This discussion was between two nurses whom I later identified as belonging to a group which I called the controllers. This was a group of (predominantly) nurses violently opposed to most kinds of therapeutic community activity and it was this kind of inside information which smacked of conflict within their unit. Since much of my work was made up of interviews and observations of these and other nursing groups it might be useful to say something about the 'theory' which lies behind this.

Participant observation

Although participant observation and interviews are separate approaches, the literature often depicts observation as the primary method of qualitative research (Becker and Geer 1970). Ragucci (1972) holds that 'participant observation is synonymous with the ethnographic approach' and Lofland (1976) similarly sees it as the yardstick against which other methods are compared. Others (Schatzman and Strauss 1973; Lofland and Lofland 1984) regard this distinction as overdrawn and West (1980: 13) states that '... the bulk of participant observation data is probably gathered through informal interviews and supplemented by observation'.

In fact, a blend of both methods is the central technique of naturalistic investigations and in the present case, interviewing became an integral element in what was observed. So as to remain faithful to the idea of natural involvement, however, I conducted my interviews in as casual a manner as possible.

The literature appears to neglect potential incompatibility between formal social investigations and casualness in interviewing. Ragucci (1972: 487) states: 'Scientific observation is deliberate search, carried out with care and forethought, as contrasted with the casual and largely passive perceptions of everyday life.'

In order to effect a degree of formality within qualitative studies, deliberateness and control substitute for the use of special instruments in quantitative studies. However, the relative success of the participant role is predicated on the ability to establish rapport and trust with informants. Congruence is important and even how one presents oneself may influence the data obtained (Clifford and Gough 1990). I played down my role as researcher by adopting a 'one of the lads' stance so as to worm my way into their confidence and thus elicit less guarded accounts.

Method

My observations occurred over a six week period and the method used was mainly eavesdropping, described by Schatzman and Strauss (1973) as 'a major source of information'. Similarly, Bloor (1980) (drawing from Goffman 1959) refers to 'backstage information' as an important source of data and Reid (1991) describes 'hanging around chatting' as a method of obtaining information. O'Brian (1974) calls the process of eavesdropping 'the grapevine'.

Such unsolicited data gathering stands opposed to interviewing and is especially recommended so as to avoid contaminating data by preformed ideas. The time periods of such observations are determined by the need to record and report one's observations since, 'For better or worse, the human mind forgets massively and quickly' (Lofland and Lofland 1984: 62), and even if analysis closely follows observations, a period of reflection seems inevitable and therefore records are essential. Following observation periods I would depart to the unit lavatory either to make notes or speak into a miniature Dictaphone, a strategy reported by Olsen and Whittaker (1968). Although this ploy could be seen as crude, it was necessary to overcome the distortions of memory and I was able to utilise the lavatory without notice since a ban on in-house smoking ensured I was not alone in making frequent trips.

Informed consent

Informed consent is important but it can vary in terms of what people believe they are consenting to (Reid 1991) and subjects often misperceive the nature of research (Archbold 1986). Gray (1994) found that despite written informed consent, subjects remained unaware that they were involved in a medical experiment. Contrary to belief, distinctions between overt or covert strategies are not as clear cut as commonly believed and each study is shaped by the social, psychological and ethical contexts within which it evolves: 'The extremes – pure overt presentation, or pure covert presentation – probably do not exist. All research is to some degree secret since it is impossible to tell the subject everything' (Archbold 1986: 159).

Researchers have to assess information which is overheard and balance it against factors of illegality, patient well-being and the rights of participants. Cormack (1981) has encouraged using unsolicited data presumably on the grounds that information not asked for is by definition volunteered. Cormack appears not to see any ethical problems provided the subjects know they are involved in a study. Polit and Hungler (1993) similarly recognise degrees of observer concealment. If concealment means that people are not told that they are subjects then this is unethical. However, inasmuch as informed subjects may begin to act the role of subject and thus skew findings, some concealment may be necessary. Gray (1994) points out that this is less sinister where the consequences for subjects are negligible. In truth, almost all qualitative research with human subjects involves *some* intrusion into their lives. In an area where full disclosure may enhance biased responses, some degree of covert data collection seems feasible especially when dealing with sensitive aspects of behaviour.

Deceiving subjects can be problematic of course but in this instance they knew that a study was ongoing even if not always aware that they were being observed. For example eavesdropping was always within sight of the relevant subjects and only clandestine inasmuch as feigned newspaper reading might have been mistaken for the real thing. Also, as it is usually redundant to instruct a jury to ignore crucial but inadmissible evidence, so is it difficult to disregard overheard material. Such serendipitous events can constitute valuable information (Burns and Grove 1987).

Taking off

I initially contacted the manager to whom I outlined my research stating that my study was for academic purposes only and would be confidential. In particular, neither the Hospital Trust or Home Office would be a party to its findings. I did not convey my expectations about conflict, nor my doubts about their therapeutic assertions. I did not speak to the rest of the staff, restricting my entry to the manager alone.

Following Sharp (1975) I reasoned that if their statements about therapy were true, then a 'spreading activation' would scatter information across the unit. There would be no need for me to explain anything. Such a communications free-for-all never happened. Indeed some staff remained ignorant throughout of who I was. However, I was never sure of the extent to which my lack of explanation had brought this about. I also failed to take adequate account of systems within the system inasmuch as there emerged 'stronger Barons than Emperor', interior organisational lines which required considerable ingenuity and tenacity in trying to overcome them. Evaneshko (1985) correctly identifies problems of entry as having a lasting effect and the irresolute nature of my problems was clearly linked to the ambivalence of my entry.

Findings 1: controllers and carers

With stunning immediacy, two constellations of views emerged, each represented by key nurses and their followers. One group can be labelled carers and the other controllers. The controllers appeared to see aggression as overt acts to be dealt with there-and-then and not explicable by situational factors. Whereas carers viewed aggression as mediated in part by prevailing conditions within the unit. A covert suspicion characterised the activities of both groups, but became more explicit during meetings and was often provoked by what the controllers saw as the carers' too intimate relationships with clients. Generally, the carers felt unable to discuss therapies with the controllers and they frequently complained of things left hanging in the wind.

> We are not good at pinning down areas we need to talk about and improve on. Too many people want to run the place without talk.

An obvious area of conflict was the existence of a staff support group regarded by the carers as essential to therapeutic community activity and by the controllers with disfavour. The controllers often boycotted this group. However, they would administer the unit whilst it took place thus allowing the carers to meet in psychological safety whilst, symbiotic like, the controllers appeared to derive some psychological comfort in not acting as mere gaolers.

Q: The staff support group polarises people?
A: There's something quite pathological about my attendance at that. I mean there is a purpose in my attending but there is also the people that go in there. We have the piss taken out of us.
Q: The non-attenders take the piss out of those who go?
A: Yeah, and it's a stand for those people who go, to hang on to it and they are very tenacious people. Despite the fact that they are more emotional, outwardly they would cry. They're often seen as the weakest

people on the unit, I think they are the most resilient: they will stay the course when others leave.

Q: The custodial people have little time for it?

A: They despise it! And it's strange because the odd time that one of them comes, it's all practical issues, security, aggression and so on and you can't talk about emotional issues or whatever.

Flowers in their mouths

I spoke to someone identified as a 'control leader':

Control leader: A therapeutic community? Bullshit! I don't think you can achieve that here. They're just a bunch of wankers! Standing about whilst the patients walk off the unit.

Q: Some people have seen you as a kind of leader ... at the secure end?

A: A lot of people have a vested interest in making that polarisation. I'm certainly for making it a secure unit – a well managed unit. It's unacceptable what's happened in the past, sex with patients or whatever. Your therapeutic community on its own you might as well throw it down the drain. You must have a secure unit. If you undermine that you have nothing.

These controller nurses took exception to the therapeutic community concept, regarding its practitioners as nurses with 'flowers in their mouths'. It wasn't easy to understand their antipathy. I could only surmise that they envied the carers' ability to relate to patients in a way which they would have liked to do but couldn't. Geraldine, a nurse, told me:

That's true but I also think that it works the other way. I think that often the sort of therapeutic side envy the people that are containers and more punitive and authoritarian, able to contain things, because I think there's a lot of denial from the therapists as well.

Something which did distinguish the carers was a willingness on their part to search for the possible sources of behaviour whereas the very *idea* of the unconscious seemed to distress the controllers greatly and often they appeared to see a trap, a kind of hidden malice amongst the therapist nurses.

Conflict and control

The locked door is a barrier by which an external control is maintained in place of the discredited internal controls of the offenders who inhabit the locked community. The coherence of rigid communities is vulnerable to

splitting however, with the formation of factions, '... each fighting tena-
ciously for its own self interest'. Whilst the carers were sometimes dubious
about the nitty-gritty of implementing basic security, they also considered
the locked system a protection against the real or imagined threat of
violence. Locked systems, they asserted, 'provided a sense of security from a
more controlled surveillance which some would find too threatening. It also
gives you a sense of confidence whereby you can contain risky people but
take chances with them therapeutically.'

Another nurse spoke about how 'getting out of here requires understanding of why you are here. Some clients feel safe because of the security
and so the security can be used as a boundary within which growth may
occur.'

Although controller nurses appeared to pay lip service to the therapeutic
claims of the unit, they insisted, interminably, that the unit should function
primarily as a secure system: 'Some of these people should be punished' or
'I feel uncomfortable. Everything's too therapy intensive, interpreting everything you say rather than looking at security issues.'

Another told me:

> How can it be a therapeutic community? They're here against their will:
> some try to escape. The therapeutic community angels. ... They're middle
> class idealists, if it was up to that lot the clients could all walk out
> tomorrow. Tell the people in * * * * [the nearby town] that.

Whether to utilise the local town as a testing ground for clients'
behaviours was a hotly disputed issue. Carers wished to do so in order to
obtain a more trustworthy reading of a resident's dangerousness as well as
being a more humane activity. Controller nurses vehemently demanded rock
solid guarantees – never stating from whom – about clients' safety before
granting such leave.

The 'debate' could become acerbic:

> They will have sirens and neon lights on the unit next. They seem to
> think of nothing but gaol, gaol, gaol. Apparently, one of them wanted
> to get prison uniforms like at Broadmoor. Anyway, you end up with a
> split because one group wants to set limits and they see us [carers] as
> making trouble for them to deal with.

A controller concluded: 'We're so far apart, it's difficult to identify things
that even could be discussed. I mean it's almost as if discussion would not be
enough.'

Staff support group

This group comprised a once weekly meeting led by a psychoanalytic therapist.

Whilst the latter element did not help, the very existence of this group polarised the nurses. Some of the staff were quite perceptive about this group.

> Yeah, and … because they are on the whole the therapeutic side and I think that it's almost a stand for those people that they will attend come hell or high water, to hang on to it.
>   They are very tenacious people. I think that the people that go in there are the most tenacious people on the unit and despite the fact that they are more emotional, outwardly they would perhaps cry and are often seen as the weakest people on the unit, I think they are the most resilient and I think that they are the ones that will stay the course.

Others were more aggressive:

> They are in love with the idea of the therapeutic community. The middle class dream. They've broken with reality. The group is élitist, used and dominated by a small group of individuals who happen to be part of the therapeutic community camp.

I discussed this with a Charge Nurse:

A: I've never felt particularly comfortable. I would guess it started off as a 'what we could do on the unit' group but became a psychotherapy session and I'm not too happy with that.
Q: Do controllers avoid the support group?
A: Yes.
Q: The group appears to differentiate people?
A: Right. There is something difficult to being a nurse. Other groups are very influential here and go to groups. Nurses work shifts and so don't attend. It has something to do with relationships but also with shifts. Some nurses simply don't go. There is a lack of understanding of that kind of thing. Some find it intimidating.

The shift system was more than just a temporal inconvenience. Shift systems embody connotations of ownership, for example the time honoured obligation to 'run the ward'. This can militate against implementing therapies and as often as not these tended to be sustained by non-nurses as well as some of the carers.

Findings 2: marking time in the dayroom

A recurring event was the way that nurses congregated in the dayroom which was the main communal area of the unit. Nurses frequently sat around tables doing crosswords, reading newspapers and chatting. These convocations did not exclude patients, some of whom would sit with the nurses or at adjacent tables. However, most patients, most of the time, sat alone or remained in their rooms. Almost all of the nurses' talk was chit-chat. The overriding sense was of marking time, seeing the day through. Passing remarks often revealed this apparent purposelessness: 'A quiet shift: the time went very slowly. Even the residents slept the afternoon away'; 'There was eight staff at the residents' meeting but no residents: this just about sums up the unit at the moment. Most are in their rooms all the time.'

It was rare for non-nursing personnel to occupy the dayroom but their behaviour varied little from the nurses when they did. Barry, the unit psychologist, commented on this: 'The issue is not one of scapegoating or labelling people lazy, etc. but why they do it. I find that I do it, read the paper: some of the patients you could not easily talk with.'

Generally, nurses occupied the dayroom according to grade, with higher grades more likely to inhabit other areas of the unit, especially the unit office.

Whilst some embarrassment might have followed upon my observing them apparently sitting around, most of them rationalised the apparent indolence as 'potential availability' in the event of violent incidences. 'The thing is', said one nurse, 'trouble could flare at any minute and you need people around to deal with it. That's why there are so many on duty.' True to form, nurses responded to alarm bells with alacrity, immediately heading for the stimulus fully alert and occasionally even elated.

Community meetings

Community meetings occurred thrice weekly with all available staff and residents present. The carer nurses were fiercely protective of these meetings regarding them as the flagship of therapeutic community practice. The residents were not compelled to attend but strongly persuaded to do so. In theory the agenda was open but in practice tended to revolve around practical issues. That being the case, the controller nurses were more favourable towards this group, frequently attending its sessions. Denise, a carer, saw the role of the group in broader terms:

A: A small number of us look for a reason or explanation for behaviours and we go on working for people who invariably let you down.

Q: You mean residents?

A: Oh yes: residents. I mean letting us down in the sense we lose face when a resident becomes aggressive and our 'groupwork' so to speak is seen not to work. But we believe in talking it through, finding some reasons for it. That is what being a community is about.

Q: Rather difficult I'd say when half the staff don't agree with that?

A: Not half, about a third I'd say. Well you have to try. What's the point in not trying and it is improving all the time. It's all about condemning our failures: no one knocks us in principle.

Another carer stated: 'We may not be the Hendersons but I think some of us do see ourselves as therapists and not gaolers and it's also a question of self-respect.'

This reflected the depth of disagreement between the two groups and it went to the heart of how they saw their roles as nurses. For the carers, I could see their therapeutic efforts as having considerable moral worth. I was also appreciative, however, of the part which custodialism had to play in the protection of society.

Mitigating scrutiny

Unsurprisingly perhaps, the unit was hypersensitive to outside scrutiny. Forensic units are closely monitored by the Home Office and NHS Trust managers, as well as by the local and national press. My feeling was that their defensiveness was understandable. It was also deeply felt although, in the case of the controllers, difficult to express. Overall, they had come to symbolise for me what Van Morrison (1983) calls an 'inarticulate speech of the heart' born of years of resentment to change (Clark *et al.* 1962) and often concealed by ritual (Menzies 1960). What was significant about the security rituals of the Ambrose controllers was that they formed a protective barrier which allowed others to work therapeutically with very dangerous people. Whatever the differences between the two nursing groups, the nursing of offenders seemed to present a gaoler/therapist conundrum of mammoth proportions. Whilst other disciplines also carried keys, there was no question but that the security of the unit was the responsibility of the nurses.

Discussion

In ethnographic studies bias seems inevitable if regrettable. For instance, I was more comfortable interviewing carer nurses than controller males. Such idiosyncrasy within qualitative work requires further examination. In addition, separating description from interpretation is difficult and reported findings do not always yield elegant explanations (Fuller 1985). This is neither apology nor excuse; it reflects the complexity of the field. Robinson and McGregor Kettles (1998) attribute difficulties in forensic care to the absence of good care-planning and a relative failure to orient professional practice in this way. Rose (1998) identifies external, political and social pressures as important and points to the present succession of public inquiries as possessing some of the hallmarks of a routinised response, a response which nevertheless has the effect of encouraging 'risk-thinking'. In a sense, the professionals become part of the problem inasmuch as they promote the representation of mentally ill people to the public consciousness as one of threat and alarm. This is certainly true of the controller group.

A group of carer nurses, however, had evolved a version of therapeutic community practice and were resolved to implement it. What this entailed was some concession to the status of the patients as a group deserving some consideration as individuals. Part of the task of forensic hospitals is to invalidate the semantic worlds of patients by substituting psychiatric accounts of their social amorality (Goffman 1961; Rosenhan 1973). Controller nurses bring to this task assumptions about what society wants from psychiatric care and they are particularly affronted by people with personality disorders who, by definition, refuse invalidation. They tend to see such people as not being ill (May and Kelly 1982) and their overriding priority lies in what Rose (1998) calls 'risk-thinking', that is, the impulse to err on the side of custody and safe-keeping.

The idea of a therapeutic community annoyed the controllers because its individualism threatened that security which they sought to impose. Yet the carer nurses had little choice but to try to impose some form of therapeutic framework consistent with their self-respect as a professional group as well as their belief that maintaining a security presence was not an important *nursing* function. As one of them stated, 'It's a question of self-respect.'

Such disagreements about the nature of care may be an inevitable outcome when nurses are entrusted with the responsibility of securing society from dangerous people whilst concurrently caring for these people in a therapeutic way. This has always been the task of psychiatric nurses, perhaps made more visible by the closure of the more heterogeneous, anonymous, mental hospitals coupled with the rise of units whose custodial role is less easily concealed. It is the ambiguous status of these units which leads to anxiety and the excessive control which takes the form either of heavy security or the dogmatic imposition of group therapeutics.

Postscript

Paraphrasing Joseph Heller (1974) '... the sight of a closed door is sometimes enough to make me dread that something horrible is happening behind it'. In doing social research one has to surrender to the issues, not destroy them. However, either process may lead to conclusions which are difficult to separate from what the researcher desires. Something told me that I would find conflict behind the closed doors of Ambrose Unit and the idea was never far from my mind.

Perhaps it is the times which have conspired – as they did at the end of the last century – to identify mentally ill people as a group in need of custody and control. Psychiatric nurses, therefore, still confront the problem of reconciling the honourable intention to care for patients with an occupational requirement to police them. In respect of current attempts to solve this problem by the creation of forensic and challenging behaviour units I am left with little more than a wry feeling of something not altogether lost, not especially achieved.

> Myself when young did eagerly frequent Doctor
> and Saint, and heard great argument
> About it and about, but evermore came out by the
> same door where in I went.
> (*Rubá'iyát of Omar Khayyám*, stanza XXVII)

5   Nursing and postmodernity
A logical alliance?

What is this postmodernity?

(Michael Ignatieff 1987: 119)

We begin at about the end of the eighteenth century with that epoch in history known as modernism. This is a period which sees the rise of philosophical and scientific rationalism together with their offspring, sociology, economics and psychology; a period in which religious thought is succeeded by secular, humanistic discourses. In psychiatry an entirely new concept of madness emerges and, for the first time, people are incarcerated by virtue of unreason, a state no longer considered to possess any virtue. It is the period in which the asylums – with attendant medicalisation – begin their growth (Foucault 1971).

With the arrival of Marx (borrowing from Hegel) and especially Nietzsche, there is brought about a crisis in the idea of history. Postmodernism begins when the present ceases to be informed by the past. It daringly manifests itself during the 1960s and 1970s when entrenched metanarratives about male–female relationships are attacked by feminists. At the same time, there also occurs an apparent collapse of the medical hegemony and particularly the stereotyping of psychiatric patients.

A philosophy of rejection?

Postmodernism does not completely break with modernism, however. It recognises its place but then paradoxically questions the notion of there being a place. Emphasising movement, it takes comfort from suppositions of there being no fixed ideas, no agreements in kind about symbols or logic. There occurs an extreme subjectivity which eschews all reference points, be they in dance, architecture or writing. Addressing only his or her own psyche, the artist becomes his or her own point of departure. Postmodernists hold that even the avant-garde (a term full of militaristic/organisational overtones) has itself become stylised, *passé* and élitist. All that remains is profound uncertainty, a context of fragmentation in which no part attains ascendancy over any other and where all parts are constituted by language which itself is but another constituent within the context.

The extent to which such representations can inform reality must surely be debatable. However, there may be grounds for examining the way in which different realities inhabit the 'language games' that constitute different areas of life. For our purposes, the practice of nursing as a multiple activity and its contextualisation, typically within hospital cultures, would constitute such an area of inquiry.

But, what is postmodern?

Postmodernists might reply that this question involves a contradiction – whatever contradictions would be for postmodernists – since they would reject any fixed or authoritative narrative that attempted to account for postmodernism. To some extent, this resembles older debates about the nature of goodness. Intuitionists had insisted that goodness had no properties that could be set out in a propositional manner; it was for individuals to say what was good. Similarly with postmodernism where, for instance, a swastika becomes a work of (punk) art provided someone says it is. Yet fragmentation is inevitable in contexts where theory accounts for little more than itself. Indeed, postmodernism celebrates the ephemeral; it exalts change and condemns metanarratives that seek to explain or justify it.

This condemnation may itself be seen as an expression of metalinguistics and, in nursing contexts, the ongoing disparagement of nursing models has become a kind of nursing postmodernism. However, whilst in the case of art the consequences of postmodernist debate may be minimal, in the case of health care provision injustices can occur and they invite responses when they do. To take one example, the 'epistemological relativism' of Richard Rorty (1980) can permit the political 'right' to utilise some inane elements of postmodernism for its own ends, one reason perhaps why the right is so ambivalent about epistemology no less than morality. As Geras (1995) puts it, 'if there is no truth, (or if truth is driven by consumerism) then there is no injustice', a comment which the 'left' needs to take on board.

Deconstruction

Postmodernism is about language or it is about nothing (or both!). Deconstruction is that process which refuses to verify any text on its own merits, which holds that capturing fixed meanings is illusory. Meanings merge into the uses to which texts are put and this comes about from the interpreter's exposure to other texts. In other words language has a life of its own – it possesses a basic 'undecideability' of meaning – and a modern novel, for instance, 'takes its writer where it (the novel) wants to go'. For Jacques Derrida (1967), meaning becomes a product of its context but is not prescribed by that context. Derridian deconstruction asserts that a text is radically degraded by the text that asserts it. There occurs a 'postmodernist moment', says Marshall (1992), where we can only speak with an awareness that disallows us from naming things, since to name things is to control them. There being no objectivity by which we can define the present, so must we resort to fictional accounts which stem from our social and cultural pasts as well as the language which precedes us. Long established notions of biography and autobiography as objective discourses are ridiculed. No less ironic a source than Kingsley Amis identifies the pitfalls of biography:

Many times in these [memoirs] I have put in people's mouths approximations to what they said, what they might well have said, what they said at another time, and a few almost outright inventions.

(1991: 306)

The postmodernist idea is about a less deliberate process than this. However, Amis' confession forces the point very well.

For our purposes, the extent to which a patient's fable is also part fiction brings us to one of those language intersections that constitutes discourse. The issue then becomes the extent to which the language of psychiatry dominates such intersections and the extent of the lay person's participation. The implications for psychiatric care seem obvious. Crawford *et al.* (1995) for instance, state that language incarcerates patients by creating narratives whose function serves the interests of the treatment locality and they call on nurses to examine how their biographies of patients may be corrupted by aspects that extend beyond the needs or wants of patients, extensions which utilise figurative language such as 'acting out', 'over the top', 'verbal diarrhoea' and so on.

Although we can acknowledge that metaphorical elements in accounts of illnesses work well overall, we may well ask, following Susan Sontag (1983), why the need to surround illness with metaphors at all, *why can't illness just be illness*? In cases of physical disease no reason at all perhaps. However in psychiatry there remains the difficult question of the consequences of depicting schizophrenia as an illness, recognising that illness models have not always benefited psychiatric patients. At the same time, depicting schizophrenia as something else can equally lead to an avoidance of what the affected individuals themselves want, for example in terms of their social needs, as well as the question of whether or not nurses would be morally or economically equipped to satisfy these.

From a postmodernist perspective, each discourse on health or illness is as valid as any other and we cannot have, as Fox (1993) intimates, just illness or illness as something else, where the something else is generally preferable. Thus 'schizophrenia as a mystical journey' hardly invalidates the suffering of affected individuals any more than it excuses us from a recognisable human response. Indeed, can there be a postmodernist nursing which eschews such responses? Probably not. However, in light of nurses producing some of the most soul-searching and stake-claiming literature of the century particularly in relation to their professional status, I think that there can be room for the *kinds* of issues which typically inform postmodernist discussions. For example the post 'new nursing' disillusionment with professionalism, the search for meaning in personal encounters, scepticism about models and a move away from metanarratives towards a consideration of clients holistically or as part-author of their own destinies.

Health and illness

Other relevant questions might be concerned with why we engage in discourses about health and illness in the way we do, how we evaluate the authenticity of discourses, by what authority a nursing contribution is made and how it differs from other discourses such as medicine. There has been no shortage of discussions about the latter.

However, a postmodernist extension would examine how language helps or hinders medical dominance (Adamson *et al.* 1995) whilst assessing how nurses extend *their* boundaries through alternative discourses on questions of illness, pathology and care. Of course the postmodernist denial of episte-mology is hardly a prerequisite to asking these questions. Nor is this century's pre-occupation with language the only way in which the homogenising powers of institutions are explained. In Etzioni's view (1960) power is only partly based on communications and reducing an analysis of institutions to an actor's statements is misleading since not all communications will reflect meanings owned by the unit members in equal proportion. For example some will possess hierarchical power and this will determine the relative influence of their statements. Etzioni imbues language with real world prop-erties in marked contrast to a postmodernist deconstruction which refuses language any referent properties at all other than to see it as the conduit through which lived experience flows.

Lyotard's (1984) description helps clarify this. He deconstructs social systems into interlocking rings made from language usage. All of us operate at the intersections of these rings so that analysing power becomes a process of disentangling language systems as people move from one social system to the next. Since these systems are constructed *indeterminately* from language, very little can be known about them since attempts at analysis constitute a shift from one system to the next.

It is not difficult to see that this kind of analysis verges upon playing with words and that its usefulness in working out relationships within and between occupational groups is limited. In order to make it useful it may be necessary to invest a postmodernist discussion in nursing with elements derived from a more norm-based approach to philosophy. Such elements do encroach upon postmodernist discussions especially when aspects of social ethics become involved. For example the manner by which any group which presumes to speak in a rule-setting way for other groups is fiercely rejected.

Women for instance reject a male-oriented philosophy of language which they say constructs the rules of discourse as well as determining its outcomes. Gays refuse participation in denials of their sexuality by conventional psychiatry. Nurses insist on a set of rules that speak for nursing, hence nursing ethics perhaps, the preoccupation with holism or their insistence on professional equality. There is also an expressed concern about how medical practice can impose limits on discourse. For instance, whilst hospitals do not prohibit non-medical discourse, they might do so if the latter tried to affirm a non-medical set of rules.

A local analysis

According to Foucault (1971), power is ultimately located in micro-systems such as hospitals and prisons and profitable explorations of the maintenance of these systems can only take place by focusing on their forms of discourse. As Foucault sees it, freedom from oppression comes from discourses that focus on how knowledge – the primary source of power – is produced and used at particular sites.

Although taking place outside of the psychiatric hospital system, the manner in which British anti-psychiatry of the 1960s (Laing 1959; Cooper 1967) challenged medical theories of madness resembles a local resistance. Searching for ontological authenticity (i.e. confronting his own anxiety) R.D. Laing animated opposition to conventional psychiatry with a discourse that partly relied on the speech of schizophrenics. To some extent this opposition reflected a preoccupation with fragmentation and a refusal to see the world as a coherent entity with proper roles, obligations, perceptions and attitudes. This quickly led to a consideration of schizophrenia as an expression of linguistic complexity (Harvey 1992) where producing recognisable sentences became impossible (Lacan 1977). Laing held that schizophrenics were diagnosed ill because of a failure to acknowledge the possible meanings of their language. In general his critique can be seen as a deconstruction of medico-social preferences for compartments rather than connections, for love of certainty rather than indeterminacy, clarity rather than paradox, positivism rather than plurality. He perceived schizophrenic language as a provocation to the mechanics of medical discourse with its point-to-point signifiers of dominance: 'sectioned', 'psychotic', 'prognosis', 'deluded' and so on.

Local concerns

At no time did Laing confront power in terms of its ongoing radiation from the centre. Neither did he suffer the burden of a large NHS catchment area. His was a localised concern about language and experience. Nevertheless, as Laing and Aaron Esterson (1964) began investigating how relationships were mediated through language, their work remained tied to a recognisable psychiatric discourse, perhaps necessarily so, and we can agree with Sedgwick (1982) that Laing's early work, *The Divided Self* (1959), was an essentially conventional text although increasingly Laing was to employ a symbolic language which drew him steadily away from orthodox psychiatry.

Specifically, problems arose when ideas about linguistic disintegration encouraged the idea of there being no way to connect ourselves to the past in ways that would allow us to consider a viable future. The schizophrenic patient was essentially the product of alienation and since alienation is itself a product of psychological discourse and just as elusive – other than to those who would use it to oppress – it also cannot motivate us. Foucault differs from Laing in allowing no escape from the cultural bondage of psychiatric discourse. He permits no distinction between radical forms of discourse and their positivist opposite. Of course, this means that coherent, much less ethical responses to the world become difficult. Indeed, psychiatric extremists could turn the sufferings of schizophrenics into discussions about the meaning of 'suffering'. In some respects Laing's philosophising, especially in his later work, could involve an intellectualising away of deep-seated individual pain. Postmodernists may respond that we cannot know what is extreme and why *should* we think it plausible that a coherent stance is possible outside repression or illusion?

So what must nurses do?

Few psychiatric nurses had even noticed Laing's misgivings. Whilst few disparaged the need to understand patients' lives in terms of their experiences, nurses generally continued in their supportive role to the medical profession. Historically, doctors were seen as the masters of grand narratives and operating at the apex of treatment settings. Nurses operate at various intersections, crossing boundaries and acting as interpreters and intermediaries (Towell 1975). Stein's (1978) version of the nurse as intermediary was called 'the doctor–nurse game', a game in which the on-duty nurse actually guided the physician's prescription in respect of a particular patient provided that the decision was ultimately acknowledged as dependant on the doctor's superior knowledge. Whilst there have been no shortage of attempts to forge non-medical models which would account for nursing practice, for example Peplau's (1952) use of neo-Freudianism, more often than not these models are the product of armchair philosophising and have little basis in practice.

Reed (1995) suggests that nurses draw upon philosophy as a guiding framework for data that they generate from clinical practice. An example would be the description by Pejlert *et al*. (1995) of narratives from ten schizophrenics which identified a need to learn more about patients' experiences and especially their drug-induced fatigue. Similarly, Dzurec (1994) used a hermeneutic approach to describe a loss of power in fifteen schizophrenic patients and Woolf and Jackson (1996) have identified schizophrenic patients as both able and willing to discuss their sexuality.

Both Watson (1995) and Barker (1995) regard this shift towards the patient's perspective as an awakening of moral consciousness, a moving from self-care to caring for others within a shared world-view. This view touches upon the holism of poststructuralists like Derrida or the later work of Foucault since it reflects concerns about self-transcendence, open systems, harmony and the relativity of space and time. There is clearly a movement towards the spiritual – healing rather than treating – and a denial of revered concepts like 'nursing diagnosis' or 'problem solving'. Instead these writers embrace the view that science, knowledge and even images of the nurse are rhetorical devices whose truth is but one element in a deceitful web of power. It is recognised that knowledge is constructed as a human endeavour and that power resides in contexts, not theories. What this does, potentially, is relocate nursing as an activity whose value is reified over and over by its members and not by any text or abstract description. Whether postmodernism can deconstruct nursing *as a text* is another matter. Nursing is something which people do with each other and this would appear to transcend whatever might derive from textual deconstruction alone. The indeterminacy of nursing could either help or hinder such a deconstruction but it is difficult to know which. On the whole, we need a broader view.

What is involved for nurses

The views of both Watson and Barker involve an acceptance of ambiguity, a move towards creativity and a critical interpretation of local events at local level. However Foucault (1973) left unanswered the question of how local oppositions to oppression would add up to a wider contradiction of exploitation. Indeed, the tendency has been for groups to splinter and divide, the most noticeable feature of postmodernism being the severance of collective narratives which necessarily rest upon what has already taken place. Vattimo (1991) remarks that if postmodernism means anything, it is in this sense of the end of history. As such, it cannot provide a rational critique of society because it denies rational systems of knowledge all of which are historically conditioned. For the postmodernists, history lacks explanatory power since, quite simply, we cannot trust the language which narrates it. Lacking any guide, the personal will becomes the only standard by which I hold anything to be good or evil. As there is no absolute truth so none can claim final or absolute authority. Those who do are usually seen as right-wing reactionaries. On the question of abortion, for example, feminist positions are seen as normative whereas anti-abortionists are regarded as extremists. We can see the hypocrisy here immediately since even a postmodernist stance must depict either view as equal. If the postmodernist view entails a claim to greater tolerance then we must enquire about the nature of intolerance (Centore 1991). If I am tolerant, then I must have something to be tolerant about – my tolerance defines that which I am tolerant of as requiring tolerance. I can avoid being tolerant only if I attach equal status to whatever view

I take about abortion. The latter approach works but only if I side-step abortion as a moral issue. If, as postmodernists say, everything is a metaphor for a reality which is really not there, then morality is redundant and I can simply suspend my belief system. I cease tolerating intolerance and instead become indifferent to it.

This absence of a point of view happens. It is particularly glaring in comic productions like *Spitting Image* where *everyone* is lambasted, or *Bottom* in which two characters, played by Rik Mayall and Ade Edmondson, violently inhabit a house in which all moral considerations are abolished. Kenneth Tynan had earlier touched on this:

> The characterising feature of hell is not that it is immoral, but *that it has no standards at all*. It cannot criticise or judge, it can merely like or dislike, be repelled by or attracted to – all a matter of the senses.
>
> (1994: 18, original emphasis)

More recently, the scuttling of moral values which postmodernism implies emerged within the Anglican Church: 'He would talk regularly about how we were discovering a postmodern definition of sexuality in the Church, but it was really just one bloke getting his rocks off with forty women' (in Wroe 1995).

Thus spoke Sarah Collins, a participant in Reverend Chris Brian's 'Nine O'Clock Service', a service for the New Age, begun in the mid-1980s. It was certainly a child of that age which epitomised *The Modern Review* (motto: 'low culture for high brows'), symbol of the postmodernist commitment to the insignificance of everything. Lezzard (1996) observed that the demise of this review represented some kind of owning up to the serial intellectual dishonesty which it had fronted.

This is not to deny the extreme seriousness of postmodernist and, especially perhaps, poststructuralist thinkers. The fact of their deradicalisation and debasement by consumer cultures may say more about capitalist organisation in late modernity than it does about Foucault, Derrida and other postmodernist thinkers. Indeed, Baudrillard (1988, 1993) provides an intelligible analysis of consumerism and simulation whereby the supposed liberations of the body, vocabulary, race and gender are suggested to be transitional into states of ever-more comprehensive servitude and control. We should avoid conflating serious philosophical work with trashy, middlebrow consumerist postmodernism. Theories of postmodernity are not necessarily postmodernist cultural productions. Yet Baudrillard could also say that the 1991 Gulf War never happened and the postmodernist œuvre *has* exhibited a tendency towards pastiche, parody and play, for example the architect Robert Venturi's (1972) statement that 'Disney World is nearer to what people want than what architects have ever given them.'

With Baudrillard, there is no denial of the existence of SCUD missiles, causalities and so on, but an assertion of the Gulf War as a 'catastrophic excess event' whereby a huge war machine demolished a much weaker side. Possibly responding to criticism of what appears to be a heartless commentary, Baudrillard later stated that the differences between the two armies involved was so immense that the event did not correspond to any modern definition of war. This is quite different to the linguistic obscurity of his earlier statement and is perhaps an example of modernist sensibilities influencing postmodernist excess.

Baudrillard's word games are cold comfort to those who suffered in the Gulf conflict. He is, however, a good example of how these predominantly French thinkers have developed a knack for formulating arguments whose power relies heavily on an impenetrable use of metaphor as well as scientific equations of dubious accuracy (Sokal and Bricmont 1998). Whatever the playful possibilities of applying postmodernist thought to comedy, art or religion, an activity such as nursing would appear to require more traditional concepts of morality in order to govern its relationships with patients.

The familiar landmarks of nursing

Who, asks Saul Bellow (Bourne *et al.* 1987), has the internal cohesion to resist the furore of economic and technological change? Such cohesion would seem to be problematic in the absence of religious or cultural norms. In British nursing, Graham Pink's challenge to a dehumanised, corporate care stemmed from older concerns about rights and the dignity of life. If, in addition to the possession of essential skills, the capacity to treat people with respect and civility could be established in treatment settings, would this be sufficient for a good standard of care? Is not postmodernist nursing, so called, an intellectual diversion from that orthodoxy which might confront injustices in health care more effectively? Postmodernism has little that could act even remotely as a moral guide partly because ethics relies on metaphysical and transcendent props more so than on language. In any event, ought we not to be concerned with the over-emphasis upon language? Language fuels hatred and violence as effectively as it serves debate and compromise. Even in its latter context it can also serve to prolong needless discussions and, in the case of nursing, frequent narcissistic explorations of what nursing means.

Bellow (in Bourne *et al.* 1987) remarks that much care is laudable but largely bureaucratic, geared towards categories of people and not people themselves. Even the impulse to care seems at times buried in dialogues about what care means or why it happens. Earlier, model-oriented responses in nursing camouflaged an embarrassment which attended the sense of *not* being intellectual, of being ruled by a compassion which linked us to humanity but which did little to establish a professional identity. Wilkinson (1995) argues that the 'commodification' of health care and the gloss of greater patient choice leads to losers (amongst the elderly for example) and the development of a hate culture where healing becomes difficult and where the absence of love breeds emotional redundancy. Carl Rogers (1961) placed human attributes at the heart of professional relationships and his unconditional positive regard must epitomise a postmodernism of sorts. The extent of his influence amongst nurses would suggest that they seek to provide such regard for their individual patients. However, the question of *belonging* needs to be addressed, for whilst diversity is not a problem, individuals in occupational settings must accept some common responsibilities if they are to escape an 'alternative nightmare of fragmentation, particularism and separatism' (Frankel 1990). Having redefined their position, gays, women and nurses still face basic problems of humanity and it would surely be unrealistic for them to anticipate total freedom from constraint. At the same time, there is a serviceable sense in which postmodernist thinking ratifies the break-up of coercive group identities and this can be useful in dissolving contemporary structures of nursing. The particular concerns of psychiatric nurses, for instance, can hardly unite if constantly smothered by general nurses whose numbers are much greater and whose history is utterly different. Whilst all groups, be they gays, feminists or carers, must share general concerns about equity, discrimination and justice, there also remains that cultural identity which defines the actual group or sub-group involved be they psychiatric nurses or patients. This desire for autonomy is no mere celebration of arbitrariness, nor is it just dallying with yet another model. Rather it seeks to ameliorate psychiatric disturbance and is particularly rooted in concerns about human welfare which originate in cultural–religious traditions that are older than postmodernism. As noted, postmodernism is about denying the ways in which history informs the present. Older traditions however summon us to act in a fundamentally right way towards people in distress, a way that we have generally come to call caring.

Viva South Ockendon!

Yet, why *should* anyone care when from the postmodernist viewpoint the very notion of care having special standing is contentious? We suppose that nurses possess an inherent disposition to care, yet sufficient examples exist to warrant an opposing view (Robb 1967; DHSS 1969, 1971, 1972, 1974; Stockwell 1972; Martin 1984; Lunder 1987; Blom-Cooper 1992; Penhale 1995; Vernon 1995; *Guardian* 1996; *Nursing Times* 1997; Rowden 1998). Part of the problem has been too strong an emphasis on the doctor–nurse relationship, whilst neglecting what it is that nurses do with patients. Hewiston (1995) suggests that nurses are immensely powerful in relation to patients whom, he says, they control by language as well as the related tendency to categorise people and delineate them by clinical groupings. Histories of psychiatric care which play down authoritarianism and cruelty are as dishonest a metanarrative as you can get. At least a postmodernist stance makes us confront received notions of who and what we are. What it disallows, of course, is any sense of purpose, any rationale which would make sense of our future. Yet diversity may be something to embrace and psychiatric nurses could have had some regard for the challenges outlined by Laing (1959) and Cooper (1967). Equally could they have confronted at local level – that is, in Foucaultian terms – those abuses which infested hospital after hospital during the same period. Instead they unreservedly embraced the Rogerian encounter movement which only served to conceal the more invidious effects of medical psychiatric practice on patients.

Does postmodernism even exist?

Jamie: It was the sixties.
Alex: It was nineteen seventy-one.
Jamie: The sixties didn't start 'till nineteen seventy-one.

(Bleasdale 1995)

In other words, do movements represent events or are they terms which intellectuals invent to denote multiple events and which *suggest* a totality. To say that Michaelangelo's *Pietá* is a part of the Renaissance sounds odd. For example, what, when or where was the Renaissance?

> In short, if by 'real' as applied to happenings we mean [the Enlightenment] actually occurred, then the question arises as to whether, for instance, the Enlightenment was a real phenomenon of which it can be said 'it' actually occurred.
>
> (Lemon 1995: 250)

The distance between the abstraction and the act becomes clear if we think of a game of cricket: the game is played to a set of rules but the rules are not the game. Lemon (1995) suggests that words like Renaissance are ideas which echo various events but are themselves not events. If true for the Enlightenment, then how spectacularly true for a postmodernism which is virtually constituted by discussions of its existence. Whether a system which attempts to unravel the present through a set of linguistic rules which constitute the present can be of any use to social or nursing professions must be debatable. If notions of self for instance are asserted to be linguistic effects and not grounds for discussion, then sensible communication becomes impossible and we have what Kingsley Amis called '... the abandonment of all decent seriousness' (Jacobs 1995: 184).

Just trying to define postmodernism – postmodernists would say that this completely misses the point – ultimately becomes tiresome. For to assert that 'postmodernism is ... ' is to immediately refute oneself since postmodernism holds that language cannot denote reality, that at best it posits multiple, shifting realities. If we are to proceed we must place the word 'is' within inverted commas. This of course is a trick but if we do not perform the trick, then we must stop. This smacks of the kind of pseudo-problem which would arraign us with that part of the health service which seeks to provide rhetoric and gloss as a cover for deficiencies as against those who are anchored to problems of delivering care and occasionally publicising its deficiencies.

Notions of health

Too many people assume that technical, political and economic means can actualise health for all; that disease, if it happens at all, comes about through some kind of omission (Kelly and Charlton 1995). This coupling of economic power and technical achievement in the service of progress is distinctly modernist. It becomes converted to a moral imperative when everyone's right to health is asserted which in turn suggests that everyone *can* be healthy. We can see here that much of what figures in postmodernist discourse is derived from this combination of changing technology and the individual's place within it. In practice, national and local health initiatives remain scientifically driven and administered by experts and one often looks in vain for individual involvement in the construction of such initiatives. Indeed, bringing in people to define problems and devise methodologies outside those of established scientific narratives is extremely difficult and can, especially in psychiatric practice, be very uncomfortable. One means by which health discussions have been widened is through the popularisation of the concept of health and especially health promotion. A positive outcome of this is that it encourages people to take up activities (or the reverse) which do promote health.

However, emphasising health at the expense of disease also avoids confrontation with pain and suffering. In addition, hoped-for, ultimate states of well-being are more imaginary than real. Such discourses can degrade people's problems *now*. In his later years, Laing inclined towards this, occupying a high moral ground while conventional psychiatry grubbied its fingers in the worldly treatments it insisted on prescribing. Similarly, nurse educators have contrived disease-free syllabuses aimed at ridding nursing of timeworn notions of illness and death. A utopian world where all have health in equal measure (by whatever means) is implausible. Postmodernist constructions where all have the potential to purchase health seems equally doubtful.

As Kelly and Charlton (1995) note, living is a risky business and you cannot always buy your way into health, especially from a position of ill health. The occurrence of illness and the patient's response to it and its treatment is what justifies a nursing involvement, an involvement based on some skills but justified on the grounds of those skills being deployed as part of an advocacy ethic. Holdsworth (1997) states that if such normative truths are abandoned in nursing then what hope can there be for a nursing ethics or any principled response to patient's problems? In my view the virtual deletion of illness in nursing curricula represents an even greater distortion of traditional values. However, some caution is needed before completely laying aside the kind of critical edge which postmodernism provides. Whilst there is much in postmodernist discussion which is frankly gibberish, it at least provides some space to work out whose interests are being served within psychiatric and other medical transactions. Merely to include a postmodernist dimension is to reduce the power which élite practitioner-groups have exercised in the past.

6   The socialisation of ideas in psychiatric nursing

Recent developments in medical technology such as Positron Emission Tomography (PET scans) have given rise to statements concerning the pathological basis of schizophrenia (Gournay 1995, 1998; Hallstrom 1998). It has been asserted that the PET scan heralds a new age of diagnosis and treatment, its pictures of altered blood flow and disordered cerebral structures a veritable window on the world of schizophrenia. Such claims take no account of the way people experience schizophrenia nor of the fact of people having the disorder for many years. Further, advocates of a biological basis of behaviour quietly ignore PET scan readings which indicate neurological differences within normal populations (Sass 1992).

And yet enthusiasm for technological developments is understandable because for the first time it becomes possible for clinicians to move beyond sense impressions when making a diagnosis. Now the PET scan provides them with a measuring tool by which to back their clinical judgements and diagnoses. It is a curious anomaly that whereas medicine comes of age when 'the medical gaze' (Foucault 1971) shifts from metaphysical considerations to the body and thus from the mind to the brain, psychiatry continues to rely upon behaviour as the main source for its diagnoses. Neither, of course, can psychiatry ignore behaviour which social and cultural norms find offensive or troublesome although whether or not these norms determine psychiatric diagnoses is debatable. Another point of difference with physical medicine is that in psychiatry the mind/brain question continues to plague professionals in their striving towards an objective value-free psychiatric practice. For example it permits the philosopher/psychiatrist Thomas Szasz (1976, 1994) to persist in his argument that in the absence of a physical pathology there is serious doubt about whether, in the case of schizophrenia, we are dealing with an illness at all. Until PET scan technology, a measure of credence could be given to Szasz's ideas and mental illness could be seen as a kind of phantom, occasionally hovering on the sidelines of science – discoveries of urine metabolites as causative elements perhaps, or the continuing relevance of the dopamine hypothesis – but with the validity of its medical status still at the mercy of contentious debates (Jaynes 1976; Baruch and Treacher 1978; Ingleby 1981; Boyle 1990; Jenner et al. 1993; Szasz

1994). More recently these debates have been transposed to psychiatric nursing (*Nursing Times* 1998) where leading advocates have argued the benefits of new technologies and new drugs in opposition to the value of human experience as the central focus of nursing relationships.

The king! The king!

Whether the medicalisation of odd or challenging behaviours can be traced to the eighteenth century is a moot point (Porter 1987, chapter 1). It is a fair assumption however that from the moment George III went mad something had to be done. Few now doubt that the King's illness (probably a metabolic disorder called Porphyria) was the impetus for a medically determined rationale for madness which, until then, was seen as the product of demonic possession. Not that progression from superstition to rationalism was a smooth ride. From the 1930s to the 1950s, experiment after experiment was performed on mentally ill people in the search for treatments. Whatever finesse accrued from performing brain operations was at the expense of thousands of schizophrenic and other patients being given these operations when in their 'developmental phase'. From the 1950s when some Medical Superintendents performed autopsies on dead schizophrenic patients in an effort to establish their neuropathology, to the 1980s when similar patients were given renal dialysis so as to wash unknown substances from their systems, the search for biological flaws has been long and arduous. You might think that the relative absence of success would be dispiriting to biologically minded clinicians and nurses alike. This is far from the case, however. Indeed, the prevailing tendency has been to seize upon anything which looks therapeutically promising whilst simultaneously over-estimating the occasional modest advances which do occur. Psychiatry's biggest success so far has been a range of drugs which are claimed to attack psychotic symptoms without leading to overall clouding of consciousness. Whilst the success of these drugs can be discussed in various ways (Ramon 1985; Gournay and Grey 1998) their general endorsement by nurses cannot be doubted. Whilst small numbers of nurses occasionally question the use of drugs, for example the elderly care 'cosmic nurses' (Goodwin and Mangan 1985, 1990), in the main psychiatric nurses unflinchingly affirm their support for them. It is in this instance that the PET scan becomes another in a long line of breakthroughs. Whatever its direct relevance to patient care, its significance at the moment lies in the support which it lends to medical constructs of mental illness.

Little enthusiasm

Until now, nurses have shown little enthusiasm in tackling questions about psychiatric illness, its nature, origins or significance within society. Nursing debates have traditionally focused on how best to respond to psychiatric distress. As 'knowledgeable doers' nurses have understandably been more concerned with patients' problems in living rather than theories of causation. However, any notion of restricting nursing discussions to a caring dimension were upset when some nurses (Gournay 1995; Gournay and Gray 1998) declared that the humanist/caring perspective of recent years was misplaced and that the time had come for nurses to re-examine their position in the light of new scientific discoveries. This was a clarion call for a different kind of nursing curriculum, one in which developments in bio-technology and cognitive sciences would occupy a central role. Central to these claims was the idea that some illnesses were more biologically driven than others as well as being more enduring and more serious.

The corollary of this was that community psychiatric nurses were spending too much time with patients who were not ill enough, the implication being that these patients' illnesses lacked sufficient biological or genetic status.

This emphasis on serious and enduring mental illness goes hand-in-hand with the suggestion that it is not enough simply to help people, one must also provide evidence to that effect. Such evidence-based thinking is two-pronged. First, it is about evolving standardised interventions with patients. Second, it questions the uniqueness of one-to-one therapeutic relationships as well as the qualitative research which attends such relationships.

The socialisation of nurses is such that many of the assumptions contained in these assertions go unchallenged. There is little new in that. Nurses have rarely challenged the medical contexts in which they work with the result that champions of biological nursing are in a sense tilting at windmills. Some community psychiatric nurses (CPNs) – a group comprising less than 20 per cent of psychiatric nurses – might work in a non-medical fashion but collectively they too have traditionally subscribed to conventional psychiatric practice. It has been suggested that because small numbers of CPNs employ humanistic counselling with non-psychotic patients, psychiatric nursing has drifted away from clinical (Gournay 1995) or custodial (Morrall 1994) concerns. However, the majority of psychiatric nurses continue to work in treatment settings. These are typically hospital wards either relocated to the grounds of general hospitals or resettled in the community. What matters is that these shifts in geography have had little effect on their medical status and in respect of nursing practice one can still hear 'medicines!' shouted through walls and down corridors three times daily. For *these* nurses, life is a balance between protective benevolence towards patients, good housekeeping, delivering medical treatments and gentle policing, all taking place against a background of accountability to stringent managers, idealistic educationalists and politicians who will opt for the low cost option every time.

In other words, whilst there proceeds an apparent debate about the nature of psychiatric practice, the majority of practitioners quietly settle for a professional persona which implicitly accepts the main medical precepts concerning mental illness. As such, calls for the re-medicalisation of psychiatric nurse education and the reintroduction of physiology and pharmacology are misplaced. The reality is that most nurses never veered from such a perspective in the first place.

The facts, just the facts

In understanding how psychiatric nurses hold the beliefs that they do we need to look at how medical doctors came to psychiatricise human problems. The central question concerns what can indisputably be classed as a fact. Whether there can be a body of knowledge which, whilst open to doubt and further testing, is still essentially fixed and unlikely to be overturned. For instance, the circulation of blood may eventually turn out to be piffle, but no-one would wager on it. Similarly, the brain may or may not be the seat of the mind but it would be a miracle indeed if even one brainless head could contain a single thought. There are some things in nature which seem to be a matter of fact.

What counts as a social fact is a different matter. It is true that the kinds of beliefs meriting the description ideology could be regarded by those holding them as facts. I recall US presidential candidate Barry Goldwater's 1964 dictum: 'Extremism in the defence of liberty is no vice', a position with which he and his followers were entirely at ease but which appalled most Americans. The fact is that people may rarely agree on contentious issues, hence D.H. Lawrence's comment that what was pornography to one person was but the laughter of genius to another. One occasionally witnesses attempts to denigrate schools of thought which deal with social issues by the process of identifying them as ideological. However, it is not enough simply to shout 'ideological', 'journalistic' or 'medical model'! One must say why one disagrees. The problem is that in social affairs that which may be asserted as stemming from a basis in reason is sometimes nothing of the kind. Rather, such assertions are serving the carrying forward of a fixed and unyielding viewpoint. Some years ago, a New York magazine published a story about two civil rights workers who came upon an old man who harboured a venomous prejudice against black people. The old man agreed to listen to them however, so they set out to explain the absurdity of racism. Drawing on principles from anthropology, genetics, biology, social psychology, history, ethics and humanism, they hammered their message home. When they finished, the old man looked at them carefully, thought for a second, spat on the ground and said: 'Son, there are just some things that I know.' As civilised people we would have no trouble in labelling this old man's 'knowledge' as prejudice.

Such 'knowledge', however, can also be deployed in defence of less obvious causes. It can be seen underpinning beliefs about the nature of illness and how best to respond to it if indeed one should respond at all. Warburton (1992), for instance, sceptical of attempts to alter people's beliefs about what they see as right and wrong, quotes Nietzsche (1973) to the effect that most moral philosophers end up justifying a desire of the heart that has been filtered and made abstract. If true, then our respective involvement in our abstract, professional or occupational settings is more than just the product of cool reflection. Rather does it point to our upbringing, the social and psychological forces which act on us throughout our lives. Naturally there is little we can do about our upbringing, all of us 'carry baggage'. What matters is the extent to which our subjectivity moves across from questions of beliefs about social systems to questions of beliefs about the natural world and how we study it.

Are those nurses who embrace positivism, who accept as relevant only that data which comes from randomised control trials, also influenced by subjective forces? I believe the answer is both 'yes' and 'no'. It seems fair to assume that occupational choices reflect more than rational evaluations of available options, that one's choice – be it scientist or writer – reflects a range of emotional and attitudinal factors over which one has imperfect control. Equally, subjective elements may influence a scientist's decision to investigate a particular problem; the particular kudos which certain kinds of research may bring or the humanitarian prestige which follows a breakthrough in medical research.

However, such decisions will reflect the objective interests of the researcher as well and it is a common error to suppose that choosing a particular career or having an interest in a particular subject means that science is subjective. We must make a distinction between the generation of scientific ideas and the manner by which these are tested, recognising that the scientific process is organised in such a way as to nullify subjective elements.

Using the data

Having said this, whilst factual in themselves, scientific findings can be taken to represent the disparate views of interested parties. The fact of some anatomical abnormality being used as an explanatory device for aspects of human consciousness when the nature of consciousness continues to preoccupy philosophical inquiry is a case in point. Some nurses have been too quick to act on this information which they have elevated out of all proportion. They have attributed too much credence to laboratory findings, as if these constitute progressive, composite explanations of psychiatric illness when actually the occasional unearthing of such information is matched by findings which run in an opposite direction.

Notwithstanding this, a minority of psychiatric nurses remain disillusioned about scientific findings and debates about what constitutes the facts have never been resolved. For example, it is argued that psychiatrically distressed people are often at the mercy of intolerant or at least unsympathetic environments. That being the case, approaches which involve mediation between the patient and his surroundings are likely to be helpful especially when the therapist is familiar with the patient's aspirations. The more one takes account of human experience, the more difficult it becomes to utilise the language of diagnostics and therapeutics. The latter:

> take relatively little account of what the person is, how the world seems to him or her, what he or she is striving for. Psychological therapies, however falteringly, at least struggle to make the person's own vision of the world the starting point.
>
> (Bannister 1998: 219)

You light up my life

Professor Gournay (1998: 41) has said 'I have sat in the scanning room and watched people's brains lighting up as they hallucinate in a way that normal brains don't.' To regard such scans as the brain is erroneous. A scan is an artefact, a representation of neuronal function and Gournay's remark exaggerates the usefulness of PET scan imagery. As Jaynes notes:

> Research in this area is as obstinate a tangle of control difficulties as can be found anywhere. How may we study schizophrenia and at the same time eliminate the effects of hospitalisation, of drugs, of prior therapy, of cultural expectation, of uniting learned reactions to bizarre experiences, or of differences in obtaining accurate data about the situational crises of people who, through the trauma of hospitalisation, find it frightening to communicate.
>
> (1976: 407)

At best, blood flow alterations which appear to accompany human thought may provide a correlation between both phenomena, much in the same way that rapid eye movements (REM sleep) accompany dreaming. REM sleep, however, tells us little about the content of dreams, neither does it tell us why we dream.

That laboratory research might head the agenda of bio-chemists and organic psychiatrists is understandable. That it should come high on the priorities of some nurses is perplexing. I can see that nurses might be *interested*; what I cannot understand is why they should seek to emulate the concerns of another profession. I would have expected nurses to be preoccupied with patient's relationships and experiences. Not that doing so would be without its problems, for instance the difficulty of defining a knowledge base from experiential principles as well as the problem of trying to evaluate such knowledge. An important response to this dilemma has been the development of qualitative research strategies which seek to address the meanings inherent in social engagements. For Gournay (1998) 'Qualitative inquiries are very engaging at first sight but look closer and the integrity becomes very thin and then non-existent.'

However, it is the integrity of nursing responses to distressed patients which matters most and not the relative merits of research paradigms. The question for nurses is the utilisation of knowledge in dealing with patient's problems rather than questions which focus on the purity of ideas or the manner of their origin.

In Patrick Kavanagh's novel *Tarry Flynn* (1965), a young poet farms a dismal plot of land because his mother and sisters still live on it. He aches for Paris and London and jeers at the local farm yokels who, neither able to read or write, seem too content with their lot. At a fête, Tarry buys a volume of poems and prides himself on showing them off. The yokels he contemptuously observes buying coloured books, books with pictures! Later, when the Land Commission comes to his village to apportion available plots of land by bidding, poor Tarry is left with more stony ground whilst the yokels get arable pastures. Kavanagh's point is that volumes of poetry are little use when it comes to tilling land but books with pictures can be helpful if they happen to be ordinance survey maps with advice on which land is arable and which is not.

Knowledge is only useful in some contexts and may have little utility if what one seeks to do is grounded in the practicalities of living in the real world. Adding physiology and pharmacology to nursing curricula might improve the care of patients. Schooling nurses in the finer points of PET scan imagery might advance the care of people with schizophrenia, although precisely how is anyone's guess when the nature of the schizophrenic patient's problems typically stem from difficulties in his/her social world.

Split values

Psychiatry is unique in that the socialisation of its aspirants is not just about inculcating techniques or even the introjection of value systems. In psychiatry, these values are split and whilst general nurses must acclimatise to new technology as well as the demands of service versus education (Melia 1987) psychiatric nurses are exposed to deeper ideological issues relating to the challenge which mentally ill people can present within the social system. As Stephen Tilley (1997: ix) remarks: 'Anyone considering becoming a mental health nurse is entering a contested field ... mental health nursing is now many voiced, not one voiced.'

To choose the relative certainties of organic psychiatry with its diagnoses and prescription minimises the moral dilemmas which are an inherent part of psychiatric practice. However, my view is that most psychiatric nurses actually do this and that the ideological issues which Tilley hints at are the province of a minority.

Discussions about the occupational socialisation of nurses, therefore, are about two distinct groups. First there is the minority – comprised of the bio-technologists and the humanists – which sustains the humanistic versus technology debate. The humanist arguments are philosophical by nature and with a particular fondness for eastern influences. This group is expansive in its thought, intense in its respect of individuals and wary of what it sees as psychiatry's disposition towards dominance and control. It is a romantic group, wise (it thinks), ebullient, libertarian and resolutely committed to experience.

Bio-technology nurses alternatively are committed to empirical testing, sensible in their views, antagonistic towards philosophy and angry at being misinterpreted. Their desire is to explain mental illness in physical terms. Hence their comfortable alliance with medicine. At times they appear faintly embarrassed by the other group's preoccupation with what they see as 'esoteric', even metaphysical problems.

The second group, comprising the majority, proceed with little awareness that such debates are actually taking place. Speaking from the minority camp Professor Gournay says of the minority groups (1998: 41): 'We are pretty superfluous to the care and treatment most people get on the ground, and a lot of nurses won't have heard of us.' This is not to say that the majority of nurses avoid ethical debate. However, they probably engage with ethics routinely in the sense that much of what they do is so ethically ingrained that confronted with moral problems on a daily basis, they evolve patterns of ethical responding almost as second nature. To do the patient no harm in this sense would mean performing tasks *seemingly* with little thought but within safe limits of custom and practice, with well-rehearsed skill.

There is little here of which to be certain. Nevertheless the intuitive aversion which practising nurses have for academic concerns may reflect their *feel* for the place of routine, common sense and duty to care in their work. This may indicate why the practice area becomes so important an arena in the socialisation of nurses. Student nurses quickly learn that the service area is where sanction ultimately rests for what they may or may not do. Implicitly they come to see that medical decisions determine power relationships within service areas with perhaps a concomitant realisation that there is little that nursing could do to question that.

In psychiatry

Whilst undergoing educational placements within psychiatric units it has become a cliché for general nursing students to complain that a) 'they have very little to do' on these wards and b) that the psychiatric nurses 'seem to sit around most of the day smoking cigarettes and drinking coffee'. Of course, such observations take their impetus from the ubiquitous busyness of typical medical wards. This apparent lack of practicality in psychiatric settings, however, belies psychological, historical and occupational reasons which can, in fact, account for the supposed idleness.

Traditionally, there is a sense in which the good nurse is a busy nurse, selfless, dedicated, able and constantly on the move. In psychiatric nursing, a need to be 'doing something' is just as pressing, indeed more so in circumstances where nurses have traditionally been seen as gatekeepers at best and custodians at worst. From Mason Cox (1896) who suspended patients in harnesses and rotated them one hundred times a minute – many protested their improvement – to Manfred Sakel (1938) who comatosed patients with insulin, we have had one treatment after another partly in the quest for a cure but also as part of the effort of rising above the level of custodian. This has meant however that psychiatric nurses become familiar with the idea of physical treatments as an effective product of a prestigious medical profession as well as an ease of ethical acceptance of these treatments. Relying on physical methods provides a psychological reassurance of having something to do. However the psychiatric arsenal is limited and between drug rounds and electric treatment lie those empty periods which constitute both the patient and nurses' day. To be actively therapeutic for six to eight hour shifts is implausible, the psychic energy needed would be too much. Whilst most other disciplines parcel their interventions in time-limited sessions, psychiatric nurses have the unenviable task of being with patients for lengthy periods and so are faced with the problem of making everyday events therapeutically interesting. It is the failure to do this that leads to the perception that 'psychiatric nurses just sit around all day'. This perception has its origins in the frantic 'dashing about' style common to some general nursing and where the need is not simply to be doing something but to be seen doing it. As one student put it:

> It's just that they look at you [as much as to say] 'now what are you doing nurse just standing there, you should be rushing and looking as if you're working'. It's always the impression you get. I've never been anywhere where they allow you to stand around if there is nothing to do: you have got to do something.
>
> (Melia 1987: 47)

Another, Project 2000, student complained that 'Spending time talking to patients about issues is often frowned upon by other staff as there are more important tasks to do such as bed making or washing' (Macleod Clark *et al*. 1996: 83).

The 'sitting about' of the psychiatric nurses is real enough although it has to be seen in the context of excessive importance being attributed to physical treatments as well as a failure generally to appreciate the beneficial effects of being with people. Psychiatric nurses should resist the temptation to see general nursing as the yardstick by which they are judged. Equally should the minority cease their imitation of the physical sciences as the only way forwards either professionally or therapeutically. As Don Bannister (1998: 220) put it, psychiatric practitioners should stop their 'imprisoning imitation' of medical research in trying to dredge up 'evidence'. There may be little in the way of evidence which can account for the nature of psychiatric nurse–patient relationships and the danger is that the evidence-based impetus may lead nurses to act only in ways in which the production of evidence becomes likely. There is a risk here of nurses becoming what Bannister called 'psychiatric paramedics' and all that that implies.

Choosing

How do respective students and practitioners choose membership of these differing nursing camps? In chapter 9 applicants and students for nurse training are shown to divide into liberal and conservative camps reflecting their respective choice of either psychiatric or general nursing. Williams' (1978) view was that, for most people, the perceptual image of the nurse is one of a white-uniformed female inhabiting a general hospital. Melia found that students liked the idea of the public's popular images of them (1987: 14) although she had some difficulty in obtaining accounts of what the students imagined nurses' work to be like.

This is not so strange if the student's image was of the angelic, noble kind since this might work against forming a view that would include mundane or unpleasant aspects of the job. Firby (1990) discovered a significant aversion for what were seen as the dirty or more unpleasant aspects of the job thus suggesting that, for this sample of fifth-form pupils at least, the angelic and long-suffering public image was no longer seen as desirable.

Only a few studies, however, have examined the demographic background of psychiatric nurses. Hickey and Kipping (1998) showed that in excess of 80 per cent of current psychiatric nursing intakes can be grouped as white British, with ethnic minority groups comprising about 12 per cent of those recruited. Equally interesting was the breadth of social and occupational backgrounds of recruits, an important factor since, as these authors note, introducing graduate status would prohibit the entry of students deemed incapable of graduate level education. Whether or not this is important depends on how nursing is defined. A graduate status by definition sees nursing as an occupation which *requires* study at degree level. At a time when degrees are awarded in hotel management, fashion studies and chiropody, it seems churlish to enquire whether nurses should have them too. Obviously, this example could work against the inclusion of nursing as a university subject as much as for it. There exists an element of snobbery whereby some subjects are seen as inherently academic and some not.

However, if a university education is about learning to think critically about one's subject as well as life in general, then an 'inherently more abstract' argument seems a trifle arrogant even if intuitively right. Rightly or wrongly current nurse education is settled within the university system although in my view to the satisfaction largely of the minority groups to which I have referred. Applicants to nursing courses may fail to anticipate the extent to which current educational programmes reflect the ambitions of minority groups whose ambitions are to do with higher level professionalism and a movement away from the everyday concerns of practice. According to Spencer:

> Candidates applying for Project 2000 courses are similar to those applying for traditional courses. There is some evidence that academic failure, rather than stress and inability to cope with clinical practice, is the main cost of wastage amongst students.
>
> (1994: 60)

This result stems partly from the continuing necessity for as wide a portal of entry to nursing as is consistent with the provision of nurses to staff hospital and other care settings. However, the mismatch between service and education means that a large minority of those entering via the wide portal are failed on academic grounds. For those who do pass through, many may still aspire to a career in which actively nursing the sick is the prime component.

Says Spencer:

> Nursing continues to draw its candidates from a wide section of the population. Many are less able in academic terms despite the fact that nursing is progressively assuming a greater academic status. Academic ability should now assume a greater importance *but must be matched with other attributes*.
>
> (1994: 60, my emphasis)

This would certainly favour those whose abilities lie towards practical caring rather than academia. However the question remains, what other attributes? More pertinent perhaps is that if these other attributes are present should the academic hurdle still need to be jumped?

The genus of nurses

According to Cohen (1981) occupational socialisation is the process by which persons give up the societal and media stereotypes prevalent in our culture in favour of those held by the profession itself. I think that a straight swap such as this is dubious because there are often significant mismatches between societal views and those of professional spokespersons. Prime Minister Tony Blair has called for 'consultant nurses' and this seems to fit, albeit awkwardly, the notion of a modern profession. Conservative Health Shadow Minister Ann Widdicombe alternatively has demanded the return of Matron: 'She was a dragon and a champion and we want her back' (*The Times* 1998). Neither of these views are as naïve as they seem. Indeed both converge precisely on the central questions confronting modern nurses. What is nursing worth, professionally, ethically, financially and socially? More problematically, can nursing account for itself as a profession and by what means? An interesting side comment is the way in which a flu-induced crisis in the NHS during the winter of 1998–9 was coupled with a nursing shortage and the manner by which the Secretary of State for Health immediately called for the reintroduction of apprentice-style training for nurses, much to the chagrin of the minority.

Some years ago I inadvertently locked my keys inside my car. I telephoned the police, and a constable duly arrived and unlocked my car. I did it again last week; inadvertently locking my keys inside, I contacted the police and was duly given the telephone number of a locksmith who, the policeman said, would be happy to oblige. Mildly protesting, I was informed that: 'This is no longer a police concern, sir.' I recalled Baroness Mcfarlane's prediction that in an unpredictable future certain aspects of nursing would no longer be considered nursing. There is a sense in which this predicament presents many opportunities for change and development. On the other hand, older certainties are going and this is anxiety provoking. We do not know what nursing is of course and we are caught in an age when to celebrate ideals is not enough; we must justify our ideals in practice. There is the added complication for nursing that its attempts at formulating an identity are impaired by a long and not unfruitful association with medicine.

That society loves nurses is dismissed as sentimentality unbecoming a profession. Nurses seek a more objective appraisal than that. Yet the more nursing moves away from medicine the more it risks losing that mystique which the medical link provides: the drama, the life and death decisions, the heroic effort to save lives. Yet if it retains the association with medicine then it risks being defined as quasi-professional with its actions imbued with the authority which comes from medicine. In areas of medical and surgical practice I fail to see how nursing has any alternative to a quasi-professional status deriving its ultimate authority from medical practitioners.

In psychiatry, there might have been room for movement towards more phenomenological or social constructs of mental disturbance especially during the period of the 1960s and 1970s, but the opportunity seems now to have long passed. There continue to be nurses who see things this way but they are matched by a more vociferous group who seek an even stronger alliance with medical psychiatry on the grounds of new technology and drugs. The working majority, however, continue to manage the day-to-day care of patients within treatment settings apparently content in the belief that they are dealing with illnesses and so dispense their drugs and assist with electric treatments. That the contexts in which this is done are comparatively more humane than before goes without saying. This does not deter one from concluding, however, that the general culture of psychiatric treatment settings remains substantially unchanged and that the major locus of socialisation of nurses is the reality of working within these settings in which they have only minimal control.

7 Ordinary miseries
Extraordinary remedies

> I believe men will look back on our age as an age of superstition, chiefly connected with the names of Karl Marx and Sigmund Freud.
>
> (Hayek 1978: 30)

Freudian loss

An odd event commented on by the late Bruno Bettelheim is that much of the meaning of Freud's work has become lost in translation. Psychoanalysis, according to a German reading of Freud, was a compassionate therapy which in American hands became a dispassionate (medically dominated) system of abstractions or, as Bettelheim (1983: 6) put it, 'a way of looking only at others, from a safe distance'. Freud had assumed a cultured audience for his work and he thought that Americans lacked the kind of classical learning – stories of the Gods and their naughty offspring – possessed by educated Europeans. The assumption is that psychoanalysis springs from a deep well, that it comes from a long and thickly planted European culture and that it is about coming to know oneself in a profound and self-analytical way.

Such a thing could not be easy. As with older religions the noviciate years of psychoanalytic training become in their turn one of this faith's particular appeals. Newcomers feel that they are exploring a mystery, aided and abetted by a guru, advancing with a group of fellow explorers along a lengthy route which demands a high level of conviction. In effect, wrapping themselves in theoretical straitjackets and collectively ignoring work from behavioural scientists in related fields. If anyone doubts the insularity of psychoanalytic education then they should examine their syllabuses of training.

Some time ago, I was taken to task (Dryden and Mearns 1991) for having poked some fun at rational emotive therapy (RET). I was struck by the humourlessness of these critics, their pompous sense of my having carried out some kind of violation. The word heresy came to mind. I constantly discover the same dismay amongst my students whenever I mutter reservations about Rogerian counselling. The reserve of the counsellors however is infinitely preferable to the royal dismissives of the psychoanalysts. Theirs is an unfathomable objection to all criticisms from non-analysed sources as irrelevant. How, they ask, if you have not been analysed, can you understand analysis? If you did understand us, they say, then you would know that what we say is true. Indeed, you may learn such understanding if you join us. Students of logic will recognise the circular nonsense of this stance. More important, perhaps, is the issue of social isolation. By wrapping themselves in a view of the world essentially worked out over eighty years ago and with its own rules of engagement, both temporal and semantic, they have turned their backs upon the social worlds of others.

Alienists alienated

Hans Strupp criticised analysts for:

> taking for granted and treating as gospel truth a set of procedures that basically has undergone little change over the years, by being insufficiently self-critical and preponderantly unresponsive to social needs, analytically oriented psychotherapists have abdicated important responsibilities.
>
> (1973: 68)

In his discussion of power and trust in psychotherapy, Strupp (1973) describes the necessary abandonment required from the patient if he is to surrender himself into the hands of his therapeutic healer, and he gives as an example of this the last words of Jesus: 'Father, into thy hands I commit my spirit' (Luke 23: 46). Again, the inference is that such surrender is painful, lengthy but necessary if the patient is to become whole, adult and free.

Other therapies also make claims to antecedents which underpin who and what they are. Rational emotive therapy (RET) for instance is quick to show its classical background, quoting Epictetus and his assertion that 'men are disturbed not so much by things as by their views of things' (Dryden 1990). Quite apart from the dubiousness of this, there is also implicit in RET a claim to grandness, antiquity, scholarship and possibly some desire to put distance between itself and the more faddy approaches to psychological care. However, a peculiar attachment to faddy thinking remains. For instance, clients are seen as 'awfulising' and, more curiously, 'musterbating'. This is where people supposedly elevate their discomfort into truly awful proportions or where they confront issues in the sense of having to overcome them. Whilst there are many reasons why one might challenge clients about this, what is striking is the glib veneer, the knowingness of people using a terminology which suggests furtiveness, wrongdoing and guilt.

But does it work?

Of the multiple claims of the newer psychotherapies, possibly the most attractive is the claim actually to work or even sometimes to cure. The cure is then offered as evidence of the efficacy of the theory which lies behind the therapy. Of course, the relationship between psychotherapeutic theories and their practical effects is not necessarily positive. For example, the inability of psychoanalysis to diminish the more crippling symptoms of patients in no way invalidates it as a theory (Farrell 1963). When improvements in clients are observed, it is possible that these might be due to such things as the passage of time for instance. The notion of the curative effects of time is acutely annoying to therapists since it diminishes the quality time and quasi-mystical pretensions of their work.

In respect of the more directive therapies the position is quite different and may even be the reverse. For example, the effectiveness of cognitive-behaviourist approaches in bringing about improvements in people with obsessional com-pulsive disorders is remarkable, yet the philosophical base which underpins this work is unconvincing. Indeed, there may be little connection between the causal factors of someone's illness and proposed solutions to their prob-lems. David Malan summarises these issues:

> In the case of obsessional symptoms and particularly obsessional rituals it is often condition four [the disappearance of the symptoms] that is not fulfilled – in other words everything becomes intelligible and the patient becomes conscious of the conflict, but therapeutic results do not ensue. It is apparently true, for instance, that no authenticated case of an obsessional hand-washer being cured by psychoanalytic treatment has ever come to light. Correspondingly, as far as learning theory and behaviour therapy are concerned, condition four is often fulfilled, i.e. the symptom improves, but condition two [a clear formulation of what the symptom represents] is not. This would seem to imply that there is something missing from both approaches, and it is high time the two got together and tried to make a formulation that really *is* complete, instead of one that each likes to pretend is complete.
>
> (1979: 107, original emphasis)

Malan is not alone amongst analysts in acknowledging that phobic and obsessional clients may best be treated with behaviour therapy (see Jacobs 1985).

Are there, then, many answers to people's problems, or does the current explosion of psychotherapies camouflage a few simple truths? Certainly the relationship of intervention to outcome is extremely complex and with the exception of the psychoanalysts the only feature on which all therapists agree is that patients tend to do better with therapists who are warm, empathic and non-judgemental.

Reductionist

The humanistic therapists seem to revel in a world which both behaviourist and psychoanalytic groups reject. In place of behaviourism, which reduces human life to the haphazard occurrence of stimulus and response, or psychoanalysis which puts humans beneath the yoke of an angry, driven unconscious, we are given a secular religious art, a feel good approach to living where the power of emotional relating overcomes all adversity.

Forever associated with the name of Carl Rogers (1967), this is a generalised nirvana within which non-specific problems are dealt with in a vague, imprecise, syncretistic sort of way. It may be that this heterogeneity is why so many nurses find this approach so acceptable. Free will appears to be a central focus for a therapy which holds that man already has the capacity to change. The role of the counsellor is to provide a safe, trusting and warm relationship within which this becomes likely. Heavy emphasis is placed on the 'here and now', a feature of almost all post-analytic approaches and there is a disdain for the reserve or authoritarianism of Freudian analysis in particular. However it is my contention that it is the *idea* of psychotherapy which is potentially authoritarian and arrogant and that it is those therapists who masquerade as make-believe friends who are potentially more destructive.

Too sweet to be wholesome

LaTourette, for example, had come to believe that the apparent flexibility and informality of her Gestalt therapist actually contained the seeds of inflexibility and even oppressiveness:

> It was no secret that my therapist found me sexually attractive and that the potential of sexual engagement between us was present in his mind. At one point during a session the therapist asked me to remove all of my clothes. I refused. My refusal was accepted, but I felt that although I was right, this was seen as a moment of life-refusal and had I been a freer, healthier person I would have done so *sans probleme*.
>
> (1987: 75)

In psychoanalysis, a patient's reluctance to accept an interpretation is classified as *resistance* and usually requiring to be analysed and worked through accordingly. We can see that in the world of Gestalt, little except verbiage has changed. Indeed, when LaTourette (1987) compares the attitudes of her (later) Freudian analysis with that of her Gestaltist on the issue of her latent homosexuality, she evinces surprise at the non-judgementalism of the Freudian. The Gestaltist she found optimistic by definition, the Freudian was not optimistic but was full of hope grounded in the experience of despair, anger, depression and mourning. However, LaTourette feared the demands of the psychoanalytic journey with its potential for dependence and defencelessness. This led her as it does others into the deceptively optimistic world of humanistic counselling where human behaviour is justified through experience and where, as LaTourette discovered, refusal to take a particular decision was seen as a denial of freedom.

Psychoanalysis occurs alternatively against a background of understandable futility and despair. To paraphrase Freud, 'I take away the neurosis so that people can get on with the ordinary miseries of life'. Bettelheim describes the overall situation thus:

> Only by seriously misinterpreting what Freud wrote can we arrive at the comfortable assumption that psychoanalysis, instead of confronting us with the abyss within ourselves and forcing on us the incredibly difficult task of taming and controlling its chaos, would make life easy and pleasurable and permit us, on the pretext of self expression, to indulge our sexual desires without any restraints, risks or price.
>
> (1983: 18)

So there is little joy in psychoanalysis. Observe also the warning about painless therapy; such undertakings can never be easy. It is perhaps its aversion for the idea of cure or for results which may partly account for the failure of analytic thinking to catch on in British nursing circles and why behaviourism with its greater practicality and less complicated theory has been more widely practised.

Other abuses

Abuses of course may simply be seen as bad examples of psychotherapeutic practice, perversions rather than typicalities. Equally, may one allow oneself the luxury of self-righteously speculating if concerns about harming clients – either through ineptness or latent sadism – are merely expressions of paternalism and therefore unworthy of therapeutic interest. Therapeutic abuses are hardly illusory however, and there is now an awareness that, in respect of women, sexual assaults within therapeutic encounters are not rare.

Serious as sexual offences are, they pale in my view against those which are assumed to be justified. Justification by therapy alone occurs when therapists deny rights to others because these rights are not warranted by the precepts of their therapy. Baron's (1987) description of mentally ill patients being subjected to psychoanalytic therapy wherein requests for their Social Security chits were interpreted as 'seeking the breast' remains an institutional obscenity not yet apologised for. The gaffe was blown in this instance because the abuses took place in a National Health Service day hospital. The notorious secretiveness of the analytic therapists begins to make some sense here and accounts of analysis (Malcome 1982; Bettelheim 1983) encourage a conception of it as a furtive undertaking not quite connected to everyday life, a concoction of confessional paraphernalia, 50-minute hours, darkened rooms and the whiff of transgression, judgement and guilt.

Interpretation

In psychoanalysis, the strength of a patient's denial of a therapist's interpretation is taken as a measurement of the validity of the interpretation. LaTourette's refusal to remove her clothes was interpreted as a form of resistance (although in her case called a life refusal) and, whilst she saw her refusal as correct, she remained doubtful and perplexed. In this context we are entitled to ask if interpretation robs humans of the straightforward meaning of their statements. Psychoanalysis purports to reveal the multi-determined nature of our actions, the complexity of forces that govern our behaviour. For instance, I may swear blind that I love someone whilst actually hating them. Even altruism can be seen as a mechanism whereby the altruism is simply self-gratification. That being the case, how can we be sure that the meaning which psychoanalytic theory elicits from a client is correct? Perhaps we can't. However, if we accept the psychoanalytic precept that the simplest of actions involve multiple meanings then the function of psychotherapy is to make complexity intelligible by interpretation, specifically by interpreting the transference (Gellner 1985). The therapist apportions meaning because he/she knows ultimately where the complexes of patient's thoughts and feelings properly belong. He/she identifies the defensive processes by which patients attempt to evade unpalatable truths or where the patient's unconscious transfers to the therapist thoughts and feelings which properly belong elsewhere.

What has always seemed to me a fair question is what is *not* transferred, what is not mediated by defensive processing? According to a strict reading of psychoanalytic theory the answer must be that nothing is left which is unanalysable, which is not open to interpretation, which is not suitable for treatment, not even the ordinary miseries of life. For if I have read psychoanalysis correctly, daily living is comprised precisely of the kinds of defensive thinking which requires analysis. In effect, there is no such thing as me. The only me which can hold water is the me which is made manifest through analysis, the me which results from whatever meanings lie within the dialectic between the analyst and his patient's unconscious.

In fairness, modern psychiatric practice emphasises the analysis of ego defences as they occur in the immediacy of the patient–therapist relationship and has tended to drift away from the fruitless recall of repressed memories or other unconscious material. Strupp holds that:

> postulation of hypotheses about past experiences that *might* be the causes of what is happening in the present may be an interesting intellectual exercise but they are of little therapeutic value in their own right. The only possibility of effecting therapeutic change lies squarely in what can be forged out of the forces presently at work.
>
> (1973: 142, my emphasis)

However, to what extent this diminution in the role of unconscious forces is translated to practice is difficult to ascertain.

Efficacy

In 1988 the Editor of the *British Journal of Counselling*, R. Corney, stated in an editorial (1988: 1): 'At the moment there is no major piece of evidence indicating that counselling is effective. If you disagree with this, write giving me the evidence.' There have been no responses to date. Of course, had she substituted the word psychotherapy for counselling she might have received more responses. Possibly the counsellors did not see themselves as treating people, perhaps they saw their role as befriending or, as Egan (1986) suggests, as helping? If so, one may ask how such a basic endeavour as making friends came to be a professionalised activity. Further, is it ethically correct to accept money for befriending or, in the case of psychoanalysis, for a process of exploration rather than cure? I take therapy to mean something which is offered to people on the understanding that it contains some curative property for what ails them. Putting this another way, is the difference between self-exploration as an interesting exercise and treatment for a debility (however vaguely defined) always made clear to both patients and public?

LaTourette (1987) talks of therapy as a kind of prostitution, the purchase of friendship. Her own therapist, she says, 'sold love, or a reasonable facsimile thereof' to which she adds, 'You do not pay loved ones, or do you?' Strupp (1973) states that this kind of talk ignores the basic issue of the systematic application of psychological principles which, he believes, must now be studied with a view towards refinement and improvement.

Balanced against this are a number of findings supporting the notion of untrained therapists and counsellors being as effective as trained personnel. An example of the latter was the Marks (1977) discovery that psychiatric nurses implemented behavioural programmes as effectively as clinical psychologists. Moreover the tendency for behaviourists to involve the families of clients as substitute therapists suggests a therapeutic competence of widespread proportions.

A new and different nirvana

Bettelheim was one of the first to observe the change in psychotherapy from being a truth-seeking process to one of utility in respect of solving problems:

> The crucial problem facing us is no longer how to manage our inner conflicts and contradictions (that is, how to get along with ourselves) but merely how to get along. Such simplification and reductionism opened the door to an interpretation of Freud's system as advocating

'adjustment' – something that Freud never advocated – and to a disregard of his pessimistic and tragic view of life and its replacement by a pragmatic meliorism.

(1983: 107–8)

We have seen in this century a growing emphasis on consciousness as a movement in search of a new and different nirvana. Arrogance has given rise to a 'human potential omnipotence', elements of which try to bring about through therapy a kind of heaven on earth that is hardly selfless in its regard for its own powers. Indeed, psychotherapists may nowadays be seen as a secular priesthood composed of various groups of which the proselytising counsellors are the newest and most successful sect.

In some cases we are left with a stance as reprehensible as it is simplistic and vice versa: 'Grow up and live!', we are told, by transactional analysts. In a world without accusation, guilt, prejudice or hang-ups we are 'Born to Win' they say. Even more extraordinary are the neuro-linguistic programmers (NLP). The following quotations from Bandler and Grinder give a flavour of these:

> Do yourself a favour. Hide yourself where you can see your clients make the transition from the street to your office. What happens is a miracle. They are walking down the street, smiling, feeling good. As they enter the building they start accessing all the garbage that they are going to talk about, because the building is an anchor.
>
> (1990: 103)

In this instance, the combination of snide amusement and furtive knowingness is particularly revealing. The following advice is given to a client:

> I want to tell you that I think you're the biggest punk I have ever met! Going out and screwing around behind your wife's back, and coming here and crying. That's going to get you nothing, since you aren't going to change, and you're going to be as miserable as you are now for the rest of your life unless you grab yourself by the bootheels, give yourself a good kick in the butt, and go tell your wife how you want her to act with you. Tell her in explicit enough form so that she will know exactly what you want her to do.
>
> (1990: 165)

Leaving aside the curiously unguarded chauvinism, NLP seems to be some kind of covert hypnosis. It also seeks to exert its effects quickly and economically. According to some NLP practitioners, people can even be helped over the telephone in minutes.

Actually, if any one element characterises the newer therapies in relation to psychoanalysis it is the element of time. When Woody Allen was asked how his psychoanalysis was proceeding he replied, 'slowly'. All non-analytic therapies claim to be quicker and some even lay claim to managing their clients effectively *because* they do so expeditiously. In an age of cost-effectiveness it may hardly surprise us when expediency is advanced as an indicator of effective therapy albeit it may shock those for whom concepts of effectiveness carry little weight. In the current climate of evidence-based care, the question of what *can* be measured becomes a more complicated aspect of whether to measure at all. Certainly for interventions to be quanti-fied it would seem that some time limit on their progress is necessary. This leads directly to a consideration of rationalist, time limited, interventions.

Freedom

Ellis' (1984) claim that people are free to escape the torments of their experi-ences (for example compulsive-obsessional neurosis) is naïve to put it mildly. Is a person in misery from obsessive-compulsive neurosis free to choose not to suffer? If they could stop the pain then what logical reason could they have not to? What could the gains be for these people? If it is a sick role which they seek they could certainly choose something less horrific. When behaviour therapists intervene to quash their debilitating rituals they resist these interventions for a while but, in the main, accept the benefits which their new-found freedom provides. On the other hand, faced with dynamic therapists, they fiercely resist all attempts at unravelling their presumed conflicts. Of course it is sinful to refer such people to analytic therapists in the first place since, I agree with Malan, the chances of recovery through insight are probably unlikely. Ellis has a point when he attacks therapists for the time they take and the heartaches they worsen. This element of taking time is prized by many analysts, and at first it seems natural to assume that whatever takes more time is more thorough. Bettelheim (1983: 32) makes the point that: 'Psychoanalysis is beyond doubt the most valuable method of psychotherapy, that is only to be expected, since it is the most difficult, demanding, and time consuming method.'

Credit is due to RET for having dealt a body blow to unusually protracted therapies. At the same time, I contend that RET could also make matters worse for some, for example, by serving to pour salt on wounds, in increasing guilt and the propensity for self-recrimination involved in its constant labouring over individual expectations and ability.

The genuine article

I once overheard a psychiatric client take issue with a nurse who was protesting the need for genuineness in counselling relationships. 'But how do you *be* genuine?', asked the client, 'Surely in *being* anything, you lose what you're trying to be?' I'm not sure that the client meant that genuineness was in any sense a deliberate move to mislead people. I think she just saw, correctly, a basic flaw in what the nurse was saying.

After all, what does it mean to be genuine? For example, if I genuinely thought that a client was a bore would I tell him so? Apparently not, I'm told, since his long-term interests would best be served by a therapeutic judgement not to be genuine *there and then*. In other words, genuineness is rooted in a care which permits one to lie in the long-term interests of one's clients. Disingenuous to a fault, the counsellor shapes relationships whose outcomes can be ascribed to genuine impulses on his part: being cruel to be kind, perhaps.

Lately, I have been thinking about those qualities, like genuineness, which are said to be the 'core conditions' (after Rogers 1967) of the counselling process, qualities which, when present between counsellor and client, are asserted to enhance personal growth and development, the striving for change which these days is beloved by so many. Amongst these qualities are acceptance, genuineness and empathy. There are other qualities as well but they're much of a muchness and the overall effect when perusing the counselling literature is of a mosaic of imprecise, interchangeable terms, a word-salad held together by a self-centredness whose goal appears to be some form of self-actualisation through discussions based upon the core conditions. Indeed, counsellors appear united in accepting the dubious notion that talking about problems can lead to their diminution. I believe that as often as not it can worsen them and that there is something to be said for getting on with one's life. One could characterise neurotic people as precisely those who *won't* get on with life. Counsellors will state that they don't move on because, without counsellor intervention, they can't. But by entering relationships where concepts of 'can't' are strongly approved, clients in truth *won't* move on: they won't because they cherish 'can't'. Moreover, this is a phenomenon which thrives particularly on self-regard and the absence of social considerations.

Initially I believed counsellors to be pleasant, generally inoffensive people mouthing catch-phrases about 'creating space', 'therapeutic use of self', 'unconditional positive regard' and so on, a rather benign group. Yet like many psychiatric practitioners they also displayed a meddlesome capacity to induce in their clients an acceptance of the social world of the counsellor. We have seen this recently in the discoveries of incidents of child sexual abuse in clients, discoveries which in some cases appear to have little basis in fact.

This is not a new phenomenon. In 1966 Charles Truax analysed non-directive counselling sessions in search of the core conditions listed above. What he found was old-fashioned behaviourism in the form of counsellors verbally reinforcing responses which fitted their concept of core conditions. In this way the counsellors were able to sustain a world-view evoked by their theories. Most counselling is about creating concepts, producing verbal descriptions in response to human pain and often as an empire-building exercise. Certain key features attend each new departure (Clare 1981). There will emerge a leader or father figure (Freud, Jung, Perls, Ellis, Janov, Rogers or Berne) and a seminal book will be produced. A foundation will be set up (with trainers boasting their initiation by the Leader). Often, the departure will have stemmed from a road to Damascus type of experience and accompanied by a 'You too can win!' or 'Born Again' terminology.

There is a wonderful arrogance about professing expertise in human affairs. Presumably those who do so live charmed lives, their own unblemished relationships an example to others. I imagine that this is not the case, however, and whilst it is tempting to say that it hardly matters, the point is that it does matter, for a counsellor is distinct from a reformed alcoholic or drug addict whose experience of having 'been there' is intended to help others attain self-control. We are witness to a group whose expressions of expertise would seem to imply some expectation that they practice what they preach and the curious phenomenon of this not always being the case.

Moral guidance

What counsellors listen to in their clients is in my view but a version of the truth and that acceptance of this constitutes a moral act. It is the more so moral because it operates in a contextual void: there is nothing against which to weigh a client's account of reality. Moreover, instead of being a version of reality it may, over time, become the counsellor's version of the truth. The client, to the extent that he/she seeks approval, correspondingly seeks moral guidance. One sympathises with the client because he/she is in some sense demoralised when not being narcissistic. Counsellors possess an exotic salience which easily leads despondent people into beliefs about counsellor efficacy.

I do not find it easy to dismiss other people's pain and that is not my intention. But one has scant respect for the peculiar repulsiveness of those who dabble 'self-approvingly in the stuff of other people's souls' (Wootton 1959). Not that all do this in equal measure. Charles Rycroft (1968) scorns therapists who claim inherent qualities which supposedly substitute for 'missing elements' in their clients' lives. According to Rycroft, 'a lack of pretence to moral superiority over the laity' is preferable. A recent prospectus from the practitioners of neuro-linguistic programming (1995) offers 'Ultimate Master Practitioner Training' with certification after two and three week courses. Why, says Rycroft, anyone should go beyond a 'modest expertise' and see themselves as the bearers of excess *caritas* or *agape* is anyone's guess. It is this 'impudent belief that they enjoy a privileged access to truth' (Stern 1972; Medawar 1975) which is morally objectionable because it implies some kind of superiority of one group over another.

What is it for?

So what is counselling for? Is it something for which people should pay?

Ought it to be available on the NHS? We have seen that one of its core conditions, genuineness, may not be *true* genuineness at all but a contrived element within a therapeutic process. If it were true genuineness it would of course be synonymous with friendship and one could get it at the pub, free. Another problem is that we seem to be surrounded by counsellors. Indeed, if counsellor production continues at the current rate, soon we will all be counsellors, and so shall run out of people to counsel. They seem to discharge from every educational, industrial, medical, even religious pore. During preparations for my daughter's confirmation in the Roman Catholic Church we were informed that sin no longer existed. In its place, there are now problems, we were told, and in place of the Sacrament of Penance there is now a 'process of reconciliation'. It is hardly cynical to imagine contemporary priests listening to their client's problems whilst empathising away (non-judgementally of course). In many ways the counsellors have become a religion at a time when a lot of religion is trying to be like them.

A nursing student recently told me she had been instructed that all nursing relationships *had* to be genuine, that she must act towards her clients empathetically and with genuineness, warmth and authenticity. I informed this student that I could hardly imagine being positive towards everyone and that there might be clients whom I might *understandably* dislike. I doubt if I could muster any positive feelings for a child rapist for instance or feel any obligation to feign genuineness or embark upon any relationship which required me to 'accept the person whilst rejecting the behaviour', another bizarre rule by which is neatly side-stepped the question of people accepting responsibility for their actions. In my view, unconditional forbearance is an indulgence rarely found in everyday life and may actually set up false expectations.

In any event, how awful to be in the company of someone who understood you all the time. The desire to be completely understood is as suspect as the desire to attain complete understanding of another, and it is what makes counselling resemble ceremonies in which one party's suffering is addressed as though it were something to be prized. The process can seem almost like a celebration, a love tryst where,

> Lost in compassion's ecstasy,
> Where suffering soars in summer air-
> The millstone has become a star.
>   (Kavanagh 1970)

Inherently helpful people

I believe that most of us, in varying measure, have those qualities which Rogers (1967) defined as essential to the counselling process. If this is right then it raises the question of the central role given to these qualities in nurse educational curricula. In the context of communication skills training,

Fielding and Llewelyn (1987) note their various limitations and Clegg (1995) connects these findings to the vagueness of terms such as 'personal growth' and 'the self'. Shanley's (1988) paper stopped short of the obvious conclusion that the possession of these qualities is hardly something that courses can foster. For instance, who doubts that most of us can feign our emotions as of course we need to do if we are to have successful lives. The extent of our acting may be in proportion to how we gauge a listener's ability to catch us out. Harold Pinter (1981) sums this up:

> We have heard many times that tired grimy phrase: 'Failure of communication', and this phrase has been fixed to my work quite consistently. I believe the contrary. I think that we communicate only too well, in our silence, in what is unsaid, and that what takes place is continual evasion, desperate rearguard attempts to keep ourselves to ourselves. Communication is too alarming. To enter into someone else's life is too frightening. To disclose to others the poverty within us is too fearsome a possibility.

The counselling view is that we are deficient in our sensibilities, a view which presupposes norms of behaviour as much as it demonstrates a failure to understand how dissimilar human responses may be appropriate in different contexts.

The challenge

I'm told that asking for evidence for the effectiveness of counselling is missing the point, which is that counselling is by its nature an interpersonal encounter where the feelings engendered are unique to those involved. This is fine up to a point but in such uncontrolled settings is there not as much room for destruction as for growth? Indeed, an emerging literature supports this contention and it is quite remarkable because it doesn't come from the critics of counselling but from counsellors themselves. Bergin (1971), for instance, asserts that negative effects in clients may occur as a direct result of counselling. At a conceptual level Strupp *et al.* (1976: 83) argued for the existence of such effects stating that they were:

> ... a corollary of the proposition that if psychotherapy is a potent force in effecting positive change ... it must be capable of producing negative change as well. To reject this proposition means accepting the alternative that the effects of psychotherapy are essentially trivial, a position which has been taken by some critics.

At a more practical level, Lambert *et al.* (1977) summarised over forty studies which supported a growing concern about client abuse. Following this, there occurred a lull in reports of negative effects and Hersen *et al.*

(1984) commented that it had become something which was simply no longer reported in the press. However, Smail (1978) provided a sustained critique in the context of society and culture and it was against this prevailing scepticism that Masson unleashed his polemic *Against Therapy* (1997). From the viewpoint of clients, Aileen LaTourette (1987) has documented experiences of sexual harassment by male counsellors as well as attempts to justify such abuse on psychological grounds. Women will recognise this form of assault instantly. In fact, most abuse occurring within counselling encounters is against women by men.

This data (Walker 1990; Ward 1995) is now in the public domain with the press (Weldon 1993) and even teenage magazines (Dye 1995) publishing articles which are clearly disenchanted with counselling. Masson's book played an important part in this of course and we may yet see further criticisms of the assumptions which underlie the counselling process. However, Masson has been called a troublemaker and earlier critics likewise have been caricatured as quirky or odd, people like Hans Eysenck (1985) and Ernest Gellner (1985) for instance. My own work (Clarke 1990, 1993) has been called 'schoolboy humour' and 'ignorant' by people (Mearns 1991; Rowan 1994) who would otherwise espouse a non-judgemental approach to life. The point is that in its very objections to making judgements the non-judgemental stance is itself judgemental.

The oblique critique

Sometimes, however, the counselling critique is implicit and in the case of Garfinkel's work (1967) it is especially brilliant. Garfinkel offered free counselling to students with psychological problems. These, he divided into two groups, allocating each group to a different counsellor. Both counsellors were asked to respond to their client's problems in one of two ways. Either in a permission-giving, positive way, for example 'Yes I would continue with that relationship', or, in a negative, restrictive way, for example 'No, I would not think it good to proceed with that relationship'. The key element is that both counsellors were to make their responses by random number. Garfinkel's work is normally held to show how people authenticate what is told to them, the manner by which they become the authors of their own experiences. In this case, the students were able to make sense of their counsellor's response even when told of its random origins. The process may work in the way that people make sense of 'reading their stars'. One could even make the point that *any* coherent story told to these students might have explained and thus alleviated their problems.

What this work does is challenge some theoretical assumptions which underpin counselling and its alleged benefits. For if clients can make sense of nonsense how much does this affect the standing of the counsellors? The counselling process asks us to accept that it differs from ordinary relationships because it transcends them in such a way as to produce such changes as ordinary relationships cannot. Yet for those who might claim satisfaction from counselling encounters there are plenty who could tell of the happiness which has come about from ordinary relationships. Equally, both groups could lay claim to the damage which human relationships have wrought in their lives. Yet it is altogether more shocking when the damage stems from what purports to be a helping relationship. In their major review, Truax and Carkhuff (1967) concluded that 'counselling as it is currently practiced does not result in average client improvement greater than that observed in clients who receive no special counselling'. Fay Weldon's review (1993) called for lengthy training periods as a protection against abuses and, of course, certificates and diplomas are readily available even by correspondence. However, this may simply point to the inherent simplicities which constitute the counselling process anyway. Isaac Marks (1977) ruffled some feathers when he demonstrated that nurses practice behaviour therapy as effectively as psychologists and Durlack (1979) has demonstrated that training of the order of 100 hours can enable laymen to be as effective as professionals.

Guileless acceptance

A guileless acceptance of theories and models, by nurses, is well-founded (Burnard 1994). Indeed, passive acceptance of received ideas has hindered the development of nurse education (DHSS 1963). Nurses should recognise the growing scepticism about counselling. Far too many nurse curricula lack a critique of counselling and it is worrying that assertions made about, particularly, humanistic counselling go unchallenged even to the point where, absurdly, one approach is trumpeted over another. We should see this posturing for 'the stupendous confidence trick' it is (Medawar 1975).

8   Rational emotive therapy

Joel Kovel (1978) refers to rational emotive therapy (RET) as part of a post-analytic group of therapies and in particular as part of the modern human potential movement that has evolved since the 1950s. In fact, RET was the brainchild of Albert Ellis and produced as part of a theory of personality and research in clinical psychology. Whilst ostensibly part of the human potential movement it became more abrasive as the overall political culture in Britain and America changed from the mid-1970s.

The importance of the cultural setting for this particular therapeutic approach is underlined by the values and assumptions upon which it is based. RET presents a rational world of individualism and essentially pragmatic selfhood where outcomes are viewed as a consequence of distorted beliefs and where personal interpretations determine future events and mould the course of our lives. In general, the cultural milieu within which therapies work has been a neglected issue resulting in the emergence of a profession which is largely unexamined as well as largely unaccounted for.

My first exposure to RET was a demonstration by Windy Dryden, a leading exponent of RET in Britain. It so shocked me that I snatched my rusty nibbed pen and wrote a skit about it, most of which forms the tail-end of this piece. In any event I was psychologically set for Dryden's performance in that I had come to believe generally that people are much too complicated for modern psychotherapies to comprehend and this seemed to be at odds with the ambitious claims of some of these groups. Professor Dryden's demonstration merely confirmed most of my fears.

New groups

Clare (1981) had written cogently about some of these new therapist groups, their idiosyncrasies as well as their commonalities, for example that many of them stem from a disenchantment with psychoanalysis. A charismatic leader comes quickly to the fore often to describe an awakening experience which points to a new and enlightened way. Primal therapy is especially noteworthy here. An institute will be quickly established plus a journal and training courses of varying length and depth. But above all, the book will be written and, whatever its complexities, these will be conveniently ignored or modulated so as to provide a simplified model whose simplicity is suggestive of Truth. The work of Eric Berne is a good example of this. There is a lack of humility about these 'secular priests' (North 1972) with their proud and insular claims to dampen human misery.

The insularity, exclusivity and sensitivity of these groups re-emerged when Dryden (1986) questioned the possession of the title 'British Journal of Psychotherapy' by a cartel of psychoanalytic groups, stating that such a journal represented one branch of therapy only. This was a fair point. Not only were almost all the articles in this journal psychoanalytic in nature and content but there was also a perceptible drift towards the esoteric, an element of distance in a growing number of them. Given that Freud had never intended psychoanalysis to be for what he called the working man, the latter is hardly surprising. Dryden was invited to submit papers to this journal but did not respond.

Yet it is easy to witness the burgeoning publication space which RET occupies elsewhere. Professor Dryden is extraordinarily prolific in his writing and editing. It is just regrettable that a more substantial contribution could not be made as a formative part of the missing dialectic which should be part of an analytically focused journal. Hardly surprising, however, since amongst the psychotherapy professions, a great deal of time is taken up with questions of territory, restrictive practice and debates about professional ascendancy (see Malcome 1982).

Ellis

For Arthur Ellis, inefficiency in psychotherapeutic practice occurs when psychotherapists 'provide [clients] with the cop-out of blaming their parents or their society'. Its preoccupation with the past, 'helps justify the whining, wailing, and sitting on their asses which is almost always the main core of their past and present disturbances'. Ellis characterises analytic therapy as something which inculcates in clients a sense of being 'even more hung up than they naturally are on the so-called horror of what was unfairly done to them and thus to get neurotically obsessed more than ever on the past, the past, the past' (1994: 25).

This brazen attack helps clarify the singular position which Ellis claims for RET. He is at pains to distance himself from those who inhabit the 'wilder shores of therapy'. In particular, he takes exception to the mystical elements of humanistic approaches.

However, his position actually fits quite comfortably within the various groups comprising 'secular humanism' for his too is a major contribution to that theology which defines man's goodness in fairly straightforward terms. For what is RET if not a strategy designed to ameliorate any human reticence which might hinder what, for RET, is a perspective which disallows the natural progress of human affairs preferring instead to define persons in terms of psychological problems to be 'dealt with'. Of most importance to the value of RET is the moral basis upon which Ellis premises much of his self-actualisation theories. Confusing pleasure with happiness, modern morality feigns expediency, making it a means to an end rather than an end in itself.

These are the parental offers of an ideally interpreted world, of our own personal salvation (albeit mediated by an apostolic view of a yearning for security) which ends with self-actualisation (Maslow 1968). For those who are demoralised, emotionally or otherwise, a desire to be comforted may inculcate an innocent acceptance of the life theory which cloaks the comfort.

It was in this frame of mind that I wrote my skit. Generally my intention was to attack the easyspeak and one-world-view of at least one of the psychotherapies and, implicitly, more than one. Naturally my skit represented a break from the formality of orthodox writing in that it took the form of an extended dialogue. It certainly violated what Liam Hudson (1967) called 'methodolatry' which is not, in my opinion, a bad thing even if some scholars find it irksome. However, whilst I am content to poke some fun at some of the pretensions of psychological counselling I am not at all unaware of the distress which clients in counselling experience. In many ways my concerns are about clients and the ways in which they may be vulnerable to the relatively unexplored agendas of counselling practitioners.

The founding of RET

Albert Ellis founded RET in 1955 whilst on the rebound from psychoanalysis. Increasingly disenchanted with psychoanalysis he had come to see it as 'long-winded, time-consuming, anti-scientific, needlessly passive and fundamentally wrong in its view that present emotional disturbances have their roots in early childhood experiences' (Neenan and Dryden 1996: 317).

In recent years RET has become a major form of psychotherapy in the USA. Its influence in Great Britain is less certain, but it has certainly grown over the last twenty years and Neenan and Dryden (1996) are probably correct in calling it one of 'the leading approaches within the cognitive behavioural movement'. It is a highly directive approach which asserts that people's calamities result not so much from experience but as a result of the beliefs which they build up in respect of those experiences. Irrational beliefs are held to be universal and the processes of RET involve re-educational programmes designed to demonstrate the fallacies which underpin emotional turmoil.

It is an ABC system, with A representing an *activating agent*, B representing the *belief system* and C representing the *consequences* to the client. B (not A) is asserted to cause C. There are also now postulated D and E categories which denote 'disputing disturbance-producing ideas' and an 'effective rational outlook'. Such therapeutic disputation can be forceful and persistent in the service of attaining a rational and effective form of living for the client. It is worth mentioning at this point, in respect of these directive elements in RET, that it is currently known as rational emotive behaviour therapy (REBT). Ellis has said, 'I am deliberately not very warm with my clients' and 'I do most of the talking', when referring to his therapy sessions.

The British version of RET is said to be warmer, less abrasive than its American counterpart. Leading British advocates would blind readers with attempts to itemise numerous influential sources so as to validate the approach. They also try to moderate the central tenets of the therapy by adopting a 'me too' attitude when challenged on what have now become fairly uniform therapeutic elements, such as positive regard for the other, empathy and so on. Rationalists say that they possess these qualities also although how such possession adds or detracts from the effects of what they do is vague given the illogicality inherent in some of the humanistic principles.

There also exists a complete failure to discuss the quite sudden predominance within capitalist systems of these directive 'can do' psychotherapies. This is currently reflected in psychiatric nursing practice in Britain where there is growing pressure on nurses to adopt cognitive-behaviourist interventions. The Thorn Initiative, for instance, is being strongly advocated (Gamble 1995) together with assertions about the need for so-called evidenced-based practice: as Philip Barker (1998: 41) says 'Nurses are being encouraged to feel they should be able to prove they have helped someone.'

Thorn initiatives and REBT differ from each other in crucial respects. Ellis' disenchantment was fuelled by philosophical concerns about psychoanalysis and the way in which its protracted nature got in the way of the actual resolution of people problems. The development of the Thorn Initiative however is partly an outcome of the question of what counts as an appropriate caseload for psychiatric nurses.

In the case of Ellis, the political/cultural connection was implicit. However, in the case of the British psychiatric nurses it is more explicitly political in that de-institutionalised patients with schizophrenia are highly embarrassing when behaving anti-socially. Hence the requirement that psychiatric nurses intervene forcefully to quell such behaviour as part of so-called assertive outreach programmes. If both movements have anything in common it is a commitment to decisive action and a belief that their therapeutic activities are based on solid scientific or philosophical grounds.

Arrogance

I had at first thought that the mantle of arrogance worn by most psychotherapists was never more potent than with RET although on reflection this was perhaps based on the assumption that because humanistic spokespersons sounded more conciliatory, that this belied a less malignant intent. However, that there is as much lethal guile amongst the humanists than in the more forthright rationalists is probably the case. There might be less to lose with straight talkers than with practitioners who want you to believe that they are nice. In addition, there is in this country an under-discussed issue of lack of accountability or accreditation of therapists and counsellors. As such, much of what passes as counselling or therapy is an improperly supervised activity ranging at best from ineffectiveness to what Tennov (1975) called psycho-battery. This aspect is worth noting when reading the skit. The potential disparity between the niceties of theoretical discourse and the hidden aggression of some therapeutic activists. The therapeutic stupidities in my skit are not intended as peculiar to RET practitioners. However, their partic-ular aggression is more easily discernible, an easier target no doubt than some of their non-judgemental bedfellows.

If this skit seems to repeat itself it is because I know of no other way to touch on a range of objections to RET whilst exposing the reader to the tediousness and circularity which is part of the process. Of course a few lines might have condensed the joke more effectively but my point is that it is not a joke at all. Therefore the reader is asked to experience the superfi-ciality and cruelty as well as the irritation.

Ballin' the jack with Mr Ellis

(T = THERAPIST, c = client)

T: So you get a bit anxious at the thought of going bankrupt do you. Becoming a bankrupt makes you what, what does it make you do, what does it do to you?

c: Well I'm not quite sure, it's a ... a ehh, a sort of inner fear which I've had for a long time. I never have

T: What is it you never have. You never have what.

c: No I don't ... em, it's the way I've always thought ... me feelings, my feelings

T: Well, have you thought about going bankrupt? What goes through your mind when you think about it?

c: Well, I suppose eh, that I think of how small it would make me look in the eyes of other people.

T: Let's get that right. You suppose how small it would make you look in the eyes of other people. You would look small and maybe insignifi-cant.

c: Well ... it's a feeling I've had for a long time that makes me

T: Have you ever been close to bankruptcy?

c: Not exactly close. Now and then I've been not too good

T: OK. Fine. Got any friends in business like yourself. People you know and respect?

c: A few.

T: Right. OK. Let's suppose one of these friends of yours came to you and said I've gone bankrupt, I've lost the lot, what would be your assessment in this situation?

c: I find it difficult to say … I mean it's a devastating thing, I mean if there's no one to turn to and eh

T: But would you think that he was belittled in your eyes, would he have lost his self-esteem, would it be lost in your eyes in your way of thinking?

c: Eh, no, no, I don't think so really, I mean it's something that happens. I suppose we're all responsible and if it happened I think it would be sad that

T: So if this friend of yours popped round to let you know that he was bankrupt you wouldn't think any less of him as a person? Is that right?

c: No, I don't suppose I would. I might feel sorry for what had

T: But you would hold him in precisely the same esteem as before he went bankrupt, is that not so?

c: Eh … yes, yea. I don't think I would see him as inadequate … or anything like that.

T: Fine, you see I want us both to focus in on this thing because I think it's something we really need to get to grips with if we're gonna resolve this problem here. You said that the thought of going bankrupt makes you get anxious and the primary reason you gave for this was the belief that in going bankrupt you would lose face, you would lose self-esteem. However then you said that if your best friend, one of your friends, went bankrupt he would not in your eyes lose his face, I mean his self-esteem, you would steam him just as before … he went bankrupt I mean.

c: Yes …

T: Now what I want to put to you is this, right? Right. I want to suggest to you that this belief of yours, this thing about loss of esteem and all that is a fallacy. It simply is not true. Now you're asking why am I saying this, what is this thing right here, well the proof lies in what you've said yourself and the whole thing is grounded in this general belief that in going bankrupt or eh … in things that go wrong generally where there is loss of self-esteem … there is loss of self-esteem. However what you then said is that if your best friend, one of your friends, went bankrupt he wouldn't lose face. This is a false belief because if it were true then why doesn't your friend lose it eh? How come you lose it but he holds on to it, that's what I think we'd like to establish here. That's what we really need to know.

c: I don't know, em … he might not lose it because he wouldn't lose it maybe because I like him a lot, or I might not be the type to think badly of the person someone if it was to happen … to me well that's not maybe what I'd think of him. Maybe I'm hard on myself. If ever

T: But is that logical? You've just said it again not in so many words perhaps but this thing about self-esteem and your lack of it

c: And that's without going bankrupt.

T: Yea, sure, but we need to concentrate on the reasons for your belief that by going bankrupt you would lose self-esteem.

c: I would.

T: I know ... that I know you feel that way.

c: Yes.

T: What seems to be important is your refusal to connect between your going bankrupt and your friend doing the same. What I mean is that the way his feelings, I mean if he was to go bankrupt ... you see what we have here is a hypothetical situation, situations if you like and what we have to do is see the logic ... which fails to link them up ... the illogicality, if you like, between them. Are you able to see this yet?

c: It's a bit difficult at the moment. If my feelings

T: Yes but I want you to think about those feelings, this is what screws the world up you see people won't think. I mean we've got emotions, yes, I'm not

c: Then what do we do with them?

T: I'm trying to get you straight on this thing here.

c: I can see what you're getting at. It's ... well it's just that my feeling

T: Could we stick with belief systems here?

c: I don't know how not

T: Sure, sure.

c: to have feelings about this which matters to me in a way ... which differs maybe in the way they matter to others.

T: I know I know but what I'm suggesting to you is that it's the way you conceptualise those feelings, the way you think about them which really matters.

c: But what do you do if you can't think?

T: Nobody can't think.

c: Sometimes at night my panic is so much that I run down the stairs trying to catch my breath, grabbing at the nearest thing which

T: Right, I'm with that feeling right now and

c: But you said think about feelings.

T: Sure, yes, sure, but I meant that we reflect we kinda make judgements about why we feel a certain way. Maybe when you're panicking, you, eh, don't know how to think straight but if we look at the question of whether that's rational we see that it isn't. Look, let me branch a little, let's throw this thing open a bit more. If we accept there's no such thing as right or wrong so

c: What?

T: Ifff ... OK. Let's narrow this down a bit, let's say that you believe that you would lose self-esteem if you went broke right? OK. Why do you think like that, why do you think that is so, what makes you believe that?

c: I just think that would happen I feel I suppose I'd be a failure.

T: In whose eyes?

c: Ehh ... I suppose in my own really.

T: And what about other people's eyes?

c: Other people's eyes?

T: Yes, other people's eyes.

c: What about them?

T: How would you feel through other people's eyes I mean how would they see you as a failure.

c: ... As a failed failure?

T: Failures are never successful. It's impossible for a failure to fail.

c: Then I suppose they might see me as a real failure.

T: An authentic failure.

c: ... Oh I imagine their feelings would not be unlike my own.

T: Is that rational? Where's the evidence for that?

c: But you said about universal beliefs that people

T: Beliefs, yes, beliefs that's true, but what we're trying to get right here is this question of bel ... look let's think this one through OK? Why is it that your feelings about your friend eh I mean you would not lose his self-esteem regarding him less than before it happened, I mean when he went bankrupt.

c: I

T: Why does it make such perfect sense that you lose self-esteem and he doesn't. I don't mean

c: I can see what you're getting at just that my feelings are mine. I'm well aware that he might feel for me as I would for him. Maybe something like projection plays a part.

T: Perhaps we could reframe

c: It's only that my feelings are my feelings. I know sometimes I shouldn't be sad and yet because I know I shouldn't I am. I suppose being rational also has its pitfalls ...

T: OK. Look ... of course there are pitfalls and shall I tell you what the chief pitfall is, shall I?

c: If you want.

T: Irrationality! That's the chief pitfall and if you don't battle your way out you ... get stuck with it ... with this irrationality.

c: That's a

T: Let me tell it the way it is. You've being talking a lot about emotion, OK. These feelings of yours and how they overcome you and so on, all that jazz right? Tell me what are these emotions, how do you define them, define them for me.

c: I'm feeling a bit nervous ...

T: All right let's slow this down let's take a couple of steps down here, I mean there's no loss of dignity here we're both agreed we've gotta have respect right? I just want

c: It's just that other people

T: Isn't this at the heart of your problem?

c: What?

T: Other people of course.

c: But it's how I see other people that

T: It's how you think you see them.

c: What's the difference?

T: It's how you think that's messing you up.

c: But I was talking about other people. They might think

T: Precisely.

c: But their thoughts are no better or worse than mine are they?

T: No better or worse, irrational of course.

c: But if everyone's irrational ... then ... where's the problem?

T: Ahhh the fallacy of the norm; human frailty posing as a common cause, we recognise this irrational consensus. That is why the problem is one of leadership, proper admonishment and good therapeutics. Why not join in? Why not become 'one of us'?

c: ... I'm not sure really ... somewhat ... confusion of other people I suppose

T: I see. Why are you confused about other people? Why are you this way?

c: We seem to be in a bit of a circle here. I was trying to exp

T: Now I think you are starting to see. You are acknowledging the confusion, dare one say it: the irrationality? The false feelings, the beliefs about the false feelings and the false beliefs which have allowed those ... beliefs which are themselves false to

c: But truth must be irrational sometimes?

T: Not if it must be, only if it is.

c: But you're saying that my anxiety is a kind of false premise or whatever ... that my feelings are no good or I have no feelings. I'm not a person.

T: I don't think we need get into a discussion here at this moment.

c: How can my feelings be false?

T: Perhaps if you'd given me an opportunity to state my position I might have told you.

c: Told me what?

T: Told you that ... your feelings are ... irrational that's all.

c: But they're my feelings aren't they?

T: In a manner of speaking.

c: Sorry, I don't see

T: You own your own feelings, no one can take them from you but they need washing, they need spin drying. Your thoughts have dirtied up your feelings it's that simple.

c: But you said the two are connected thoughts and feelings.

T: Interconnected and separate.

c: Separate?

T: Of course, it's very simple. They're connected when we experience them but not always when we discuss them. Retrospective Rationality I call it.

c: Indeed, for a while I had thought …

T: I thought that we were finding our way out here now I'm not so sure. Look, why are you here? Let me tell

c: I'm worried about … I don't know

T: You're trying to untangle to find your way out.

c: I want to find myself out.

T: Then why not look at it rationally? Why indulge in all of this stuff when you could be reshaping your lifestyle. Why wallow in make-believe anxiety when there's a sane world all around you. There's a history of rational thought, you know, waiting to be tapped into. You know I find it sad to watch people who have lost, huh, maybe never even acquired, correct perspectives on the world. Boy … this irrationality; the compulsion of the masses; silly people going around thinking they can make their own way in life as if they ought to be this that or the other. Goodness some folk actually believe they're obligated to others! Look at you. You're obligated to nothing more than a belief in silliness, a silly feeling as you call it, your feeling silly. You've no respect for rational thought have you, coming on like some dumbo. Let's shape up here, I mean let's go! Let's be sensible here!

c: I'm trying to be sensible.

T: Good, then maybe it's not as oily as I thought.

c: Sorry?

T: Let's try again. Why are you saying you're sorry? Sorry isn't a rational thing to say.

c: But I am sorry. Can't you see I'm sorry?

T: In fact, no.

9   1999

A nursing odyssey?

Let me put my cards on the table. I was against Project 2000 from the start, partly because it offered little to psychiatric nurses and partly because it seemed little more than a mechanism by which general nurses could work through the crisis of identity with which they had been struggling since the mid-1970s. Clearly a unified profession would bolster professional status more than, say, a situation where any sub-group, for example mental nurses, might claim a separate identity. To begin with, this would dent claims that there are intrinsic elements which characterise nursing as a unique activity. An independent psychiatric profession would damage such a claim on several levels. For instance it could hardly be based on a definition of nursing, for what would be the point of that if nursing was precisely what the sub-group was separating from? The breakaway group would have to define itself in a way which would give it the rudiments of a new non-nursing identity. It is one of the mysteries of nursing history that psychiatric nurses have not done this, that they have opted instead to remain part of the wider nursing fraternity and done so, at times, with considerable deliberation. On the occasion when a government committee (Jay 1979) recommended the abolition of mental handicap nursing the nurses concerned robustly campaigned against such a change and they have generally retained their commitment to a unified profession ever since.

A united profession

The main factor which underpins unification is medicine. You might think that this applies to general nurses only – even if the major spokespersons of this particular branch vigorously deny it – but you would be wrong. The fact is that the overwhelming majority of psychiatric nurses subscribe to a medical conception of mental disturbance. They accept, with re-invented enthusiasm it seems (Gournay 1995), a diagnostic framework which reflects medical thinking. Ironically, it has been general nurses who have wrestled with the problem of identity, to such an extent that they have evolved a stance supposedly based on a holistic rather than a medical model. Of course, one could explain general nursing's preoccupation with identity as stemming from their necessarily close proximity to doctors. Such an explanation is complex, however. For some, the profession's leaders perhaps, the relationship with medicine leaves no room for autonomous status and since an identity within medicine is ruled out so must they look elsewhere. For the rank and file, who work with doctors each day, the link with medical practice is as natural as it is necessary. For psychiatric nurses, the situation is roughly similar albeit, implicitly, it is recognised by many that the relationship with psychiatric medicine is nowhere near as necessary and that non-medical interventions with patients are actually feasible.

It is true that a number of psychiatric nurses employ alternative concepts of mental illness but they are a minority and, in any event, their views are usually looked upon sceptically by the majority. This is hardly surprising if you consider that the occupational consequences of changing medical concepts of mental illness would be considerable. That being the case, you might ask why the wholesale adoption by nurse educationalists of holistic philosophies has not brought about such dire consequences. The reason in my view is because this holistic 'revolution' in general nursing is a façade and that these nurses continue to support medical practice. The fact is, as the Council of Deans and Heads of UK Faculties state (1998: 3): 'The United Kingdom still prepares most of its nurses to work in hospitals', as if it could do anything else without the consent and radical re-orientation of medical practitioners.

The university

Project 2000 is about professing nursing. In no way does it attempt to alter conceptions of illness. At most, one can say that it aims to prepare practitioners for the community rather than for hospital wards. To that end, Project 2000 courses place unusual emphasis on health rather than on illness. Whilst their educational programmes have moved away from concepts of illness and hospital treatments, this has resulted in the discrepancy of nurses being required to attend to people's illnesses. Educational programmes are now delivered within the university system, often at quite a distance from traditional hospital bases. The real meaning of such moves, however, is that they serve to further increase existing divisions between academic and clinical concerns. It is an anomaly, given the long-standing recognition of a theory-practice divide in nursing, that Project 2000 should proceed as if this divide did not exist. This has resulted in a preoccupation with theoretical formulations and curriculum design which is only gradually crumbling beneath the increasing perplexity of service providers that the practicalities of care are not being met.

That the founders of Project 2000 could also conceive of medical, surgical, paediatric and mental health nursing without examining whether qualitative as well as practical differences existed between them is remarkable. On the contrary, a key element in Project 2000 courses was the inclusion of a common foundation programme in which nurses would be exposed to material deemed to be intrinsically valuable to all. What this involved of course was a reduction in material which could be seen as intrinsic to particular branches of nursing.

Against the common foundation

In 1988 I discovered an Attitude to Treatment Questionnaire (ATQ) capable of differentiating between psychologically and practically minded people in respect of patient's treatments. The test was a twenty-eight item instrument which had been standardised on different groups in medical and psychiatric practice (Caine *et al.* 1982). Specifically, it had been used by Shanley (1981) and Gournay (1986) with a view to establishing nurses' attitudes towards different styles of treatments. The results of these studies intrigued me and I began to use the ATQ extensively (Clarke 1989, 1991). In general, I concluded that it did indeed differentiate in the stated manner. Some time later another questionnaire, the Wilson–Patterson Attitude Inventory (WPAI) (Wilson 1975), caught my interest. This inventory sought to determine people's attitudes across a wide range of social issues. Widespread usage of this test showed it capable of mapping out people's social attitudes along a continuum ranging from conservatism to liberalism.

I was now in possession of two tests which separated people along two continuums: conservatism/liberalism in relation to social life, and psychological versus practical-mindedness in respect of attitudes to treatments. Using these tests with various (pre-Project 2000) student groups I discovered that psychiatric students showed more liberal attitudes to treatments than their general colleagues, a difference which persisted through training. Because the students in this study were already in training when assessed, the influence of their respective – still separate – nursing schools might have inspired them to see things in particular ways. Therefore it was decided to assess applicants who were as yet uncontaminated by professional input (Clarke 1991). These applicants were also found to show differences in respect of their choice of speciality with general nursing applicants being more reserved and more formal in their attitudes towards treatments. These studies confirmed earlier work so that a pattern was emerging with findings consistently replicated across several groups.

As stated, a key assumption underpinning Project 2000 thinking was that principles existed, mainly centring on concepts of holism, which applied to all nursing practice. This is the key element of Project 2000 because without it there arises the possibility of qualitative factors which fundamentally distinguish psychiatric and general nurses. Because such a split would inflict untold damage on the holistic and thus common foundation presumptions of Project 2000 programmes, anything which supports such differences would be strenuously denied. My desire to show that such differences existed led to my combining both tests, for if the ATQ and WPAI findings positively correlated, then one could conclude that attitudes to treatment were a reflection of broader social attitudes. In other words, choosing a nursing speciality was not an external, objective act but instead a reflection of a person's core values. I anticipated that educational planners would include some of these findings in their deliberations particularly in respect of the supposed commonalties within nursing. However, little notice was taken of this work.

Applicants and students: some evidence

In his *History of Mental Health Nursing* (1993) Peter Nolan charts the United Kingdom Central Council's (1986) objectives in introducing Project 2000:

1   To win an equal status for nurses with other groups undertaking vocational education.
2   To halt the practice of students becoming immersed in hospital cultures.
3   To enable nurse education to obtain academic validation by aligning it with Institutes of Higher Education.
4   To shift the emphasis on to health promotion and illness prevention.

It was assumed that fewer nurses would actually qualify under this system than under the older apprenticeship system and that hand in hand with this would occur the added problem of supernumerary student status leading to a further loss of service hours. To compensate for these losses, an army of trained support workers was proposed who would supposedly carry out the basic nursing care previously provided by salaried students. Some of these problems have remained unresolved. For example, the supernumerary status accorded to students was interpreted in very diverse ways, especially in settings where the army of support workers never arrived. In other instances, as Hart (1994: 162) observes, large numbers of untrained staff 'are not simply replacing the students lost, but in many cases, the qualified nurses they were previously working alongside'. The picture is thus both confused, variable and at the mercy both of particular Health Trusts and general demands on the health service.

Change from within?

There can be no doubt that considerable pressure came from within the nursing profession to bring about the Project 2000 scheme. This was not a universal scheme in its specifics and the amalgamated nursing schools (which quickly became constituent parts of universities) embarked upon their own variations of it albeit conforming to broad principles amongst which of course was the common foundation programme (CFP) followed by a second half comprising the student's branch programme. Much of this programme would reflect point 4 of the UKCC's objectives (see above) where the emphasis would be on health issues and not illness. Significant, also, was the health-centred holistic philosophy which underpinned the changes and which for many were a cardinal rationale for introducing Project 2000 in the first place.

The preoccupation with health was apposite. The first London Marathon had been run on 29 March 1981 and practically every town in Britain had its 'fun run' by the close of the decade. By 1986, when the UKCC published *Project 2000: A New Preparation for Practice*, prevention was in the air with what felt like hourly advice on eating, drinking and smoking. Low cholesterol levels were suddenly in vogue and jogging seemed ubiquitous. Yet demand for NHS medical services *increased*. Day patients increased by 90 per cent since 1979 with a concomitant increase in in-patient care of 40 per cent (Hart 1994). Waiting lists lengthened and government money persistently found its way, as it continues to do, into shoring up hospital and other medical treatment centres.

However, the problem for mental health is that although much is known about what causes heart attacks and avoidance procedures are relatively clear cut, schizophrenia has a fixed incidence of about 1 per cent across different populations and unlike heart disease discussions about its causative factors are a *very* contentious business. Further, there is little that can be done to prevent schizophrenia. What this means is that the health needs of psychiatrically ill people, and particularly the question of prevention, constitute qualitatively different kinds of problems to those confronting physical medicine and this is another reason why common foundation programmes are missing the point.

History

Nolan (1993) compared these programmes to the common preparation (preliminary) programmes of the pre-1970s and in this he is partly right. However, the older common programmes were shorter than the present ones. More importantly they did not posit a collective philosophy aimed at defining nursing. In addition, students in the older schemes remained in close proximity, geographically, to their hospital patients. In contrast, the campuses which currently house nursing institutes – typically these tend to be the asphalt jungle colleges constructed in the 1960s – are bereft of patients and hamstrung by their deliverance of a whole person psychology and health promotion schemes which many students experience as alienating. As Williamson, a student nurse, stated:

> I am constantly frustrated by the lack of practical nursing experience I am gaining. Weeks are wasted in lectures given by those who are no longer bedside nurses but who seem to rejoice in the use of sociological

jargon. I want to learn to care for sick patients but, almost at the end of my course, this is simply not happening.

(1998: 32)

This move into higher education could be seen as a symbolic shift away from considerations of pathology/illness towards newer concepts of prevention and health promotion. However, such a conclusion would depend on the extent to which nursing schools had integrated into their respective universities or if, indeed, they had merely *joined* the universities. I am not suggesting that nurse education should model itself on university courses. Significant differences exist between nursing and university-style courses. Student nurses are remunerated separately to ordinary college students and the organisation and delivery of nursing courses continues to be teacher-centred and didactic in nature. For the foreseeable future, Project 2000 courses would continue to be delivered by lecturers whose socialisation had been into the old nurse training schools. If true, then this might create tension, inasmuch as these teachers would now be required to teach a new psycho-social curriculum, but without letting go of the ideology of general nurse training schools with their emphasis on implementing received ideas (Robbins 1963) and their inability to permit self-directed learning in their students.

When push came to shove, the psychiatric nurses were either unable or unwilling to carve out a destiny for themselves independent of the Project 2000 change. Whatever their initial expectations might have been they would soon become disenchanted on a variety of fronts. In particular, Jowett *et al.* (1994), McIntegart (1990) and White *et al.* (1994) noted the persistent complaint of common foundation programmes being virtually swamped by general nursing ideology. Whether intentional or not, the dead weight of general nursing – partly a question of numbers but also a question of imagery, snobbery and sheer historical ascendancy – meant that the subject matter of common foundation schemes would be unduly biased towards them.

Having said this, the inclusion of psychological and sociological subject matter caused some students to express surprise at being asked to supply written work on transactional analysis or repertory grid theory. However, this is only part of the problem. I believe that psycho-social topics were seized upon often without any real understanding of how they might fit within nursing practice. There was a feeling that social sciences ought to be included – it made more sense of the drive for a universal profession – but without a true understanding of how this material might influence the practice of nursing or even the delivery of the courses of which they were now ostensibly a part. For example, I surveyed fifteen university-based nursing institutes and was informed by the majority that they either employed a register of attendance or random checks to ensure attendance. Whilst most higher education courses have core units which require completion for a successful outcome to occur, the taking of head counts in a university department other than nursing would surely be unlikely.

Needs must

British nursing had had little choice but to opt for a university-based curriculum. The influence from the United States and other European countries could no longer be resisted. Of course, there is a wider picture involving the changing character of British occupational and educational mobility and nurses, increasingly resentful of their historical dependence on medicine, can hardly avoid these wider social influences. The truth is that nurses had become sensitive to an occupational role that cast them in a subservient relationship to another profession. Whilst the nature of role *relationships* within work places had flattened over time and nurses had long ceased to be subservient in any slavish sense, the point is that whatever the cordiality of professional work relationships, medical *judgements* – even if arrived at through a multi-professional process – would remain final.

Nurses wishing to challenge this construct clearly saw holistic psychology as a God-send since it enabled them to develop a whole person response as opposed to what they saw as the narrowness of the medical model. The latter had come to be seen as a slightly derogatory way of saying that doctors' preoccupation with physical treatments somehow excluded them from membership of the caring professions. Whether the medical profession resent being outside this caring fraternity is anyone's guess. I imagine they suffer a mild irritation albeit their authority proceeds apace, intact.

Then and now

Time will tell whether post Project 2000 nurses will continue to complement medical authority and if they do, by which curriculum they acquire the wherewithal to do so. Official curricula are not always the best indicator of practice and, in many cases, official courses may not satisfy the demands of professional practice. Hart (1994) notes that service managers distrust educationalists with their idealistic and impracticable ideas whilst the educationalists claim that nursing's future depends on a theory-based education. Thus has the ages-old divide between theory and practice rapidly re-emerged and been exacerbated by Project 2000 schemes. Part of the problem is that the framers of Project 2000 envisaged a nursing curriculum which had as its outcome forms of community practice and especially health promotion. Precisely what they had in mind, given the experience of trying to care for psychiatric patients in the community, remains a mystery. In any event, we now have a nursing curriculum which appears to address one set of issues and a hospital practice which tries to cope with another. The result is that students find little in hospital wards which corresponds to the versions of reality picked up in their classrooms. In some cases the disparity may be alarming. Mort (1996), for instance, documented the outrageous behaviour of a doctor apparently with the full complicity of nursing staff. Her report suggests that in some places at least, little may have changed at all. Here was a nursing staff unable to prevent boorish behaviour within their 'caring regime', apparently unwilling to do so because the perpetrator 'was a good doctor'.

Separation

Splitting nurse education from the NHS has meant an even greater decline in the relationship and mutual influence of education and practice. As such, the likelihood of service providers developing their own courses must be a possibility. These might not amount to fully accredited courses but provide basic task training designed to plug the gaps not met by formal, academic preparations. Add to this the common knowledge that many Project 2000 students – all unsalaried of course – are moonlighting in nursing homes and you have the reality of nursing skills being acquired with little curriculum control at all. Actually moonlighting outside the system, with its 'picking it up as you go along' style of learning, is redolent of much older styles of nurse training and is exactly what the Project 2000 innovation sought to replace.

One way around this theory/practice divide has been the suggestion of a one year, probationary period after qualification. This supposedly would constitute a period of consolidation, honing of skills and so forth. It also has the added attraction that it looks like something which doctors do, a kind of internship prior to taking up the reins of care. However, such a change contains within it a potential for exploitation. Under what level of grading for instance would the nurse operate during her probationary year? Is it not the case that they might occasionally be required to take on the obligations of staff nurse when needs must? Further, as Rogers (1998) states, if the profession is turning out nurses who are unfit to practice, then adding a fourth year is not going to help matters. In effect, experimenting with the status of newly qualified nurses is an avoidance of the deficiencies of Project 2000 schemes.

Educational research

The manner by which different investigative teams have *reacted* to their findings (which tend to be similar in different reports) is itself an interesting topic. Several teams have examined the progress of Project 2000 courses and I now propose to look at some of their results. Maben and Macleod Clark (1998), for instance, note that the first graduates from Project 2000 style courses would have started work as staff nurses in 1992. These writers accept that transitional problems do occur but that these do not differ significantly from the types of problem experienced by pre Project 2000 cohorts.

According to Maben and Macleod Clark, Project 2000 qualifiers found it difficult to communicate with others, to break bad news for instance. They were sometimes stressed out and often frightened. The nature of some clients' problems, such as suicide, increased workloads and a perceptible lack of support left many of these nurses tired and with a corresponding loss of social life. Interestingly, few of the problems reported by Maben and Macleod Clark had to do with issues of academia but were more related to interpersonal and practical aspects of care.

This study also revealed a degree of prejudice against Project 2000 courses. A number of key terms seemed particularly loaded in their capacity to arouse older nurses' suspicions about the new courses. For one thing, the phrase supernumerary seemed to bring out the worst in some and there were frequent complaints at the notion of unoccupied students. The concept of the autonomous student, freed from the tyranny of shift systems and under pressure to think critically by an educational élite was to prove rather difficult for some.

Handmaidens

The interview data which supports the Maben and Macleod Clark study (1998: 148) is enlightening not just in respect of Project 2000 but in what it says about the relative positions of holism and medicine. For example, a new staff nurse stated:

> I am not a doctor's handmaiden thank you very much. I am a person in practice who is – what I do and what I say and what I know I say because I am a professional, and because I am a nurse. I find it very stressful when certain doctors – not all doctors, some are brilliant – but certain doctors say 'Get me so-and-so's notes will you?' I'm sorry, no I won't.

It is not that Maben and Macleod Clark's comment (1998: 148) that 'Some doctors, it seems, are unwilling to regard nurses as educated professionals who are entitled to an opinion, and instead prefer to see them as handmaidens' is wrong. It is that it is wide of the mark in terms of what actually matters. What these doctors are guilty of is a violation of *social* norms as they now apply to doctor–nurse relationships. Whilst in the past nurses might have had to endure a handmaiden role, we have had for some time now an egalitarian influence on the medical workplace which is as strong as any other. Having said that, doctor–nurse interactions continue to operate within a professional structure in which each are differently accountable by society. Matters have changed in respect of nurses' entirely proper refusal to fetch and carry for doctors. However, this says little about their relative status to medicine inasmuch as the social etiquette of relationships does not necessarily imply a nursing influence on medical *judgements*. Changes in the social organisation of professional relationships hardly constitutes criteria by which nursing can redefine itself as an autonomous body with power to influence medical judgements. Yet some are prepared to argue that a genuine shift in professional status has taken place in nursing. According to Macleod Clark *et al.* (1996) the 'independence, assertiveness and autonomy' of the new nurse contrasts with the failings of what Beardshaw and Robinson (1990) call 'the insecure, ritual-bound, task-orientated one of the past'. The 'compliant, willing, caring and dedicated angel who has no career ambitions' (Bridges 1990) is replaced by the 'flexible, adaptable, critically analytic and autonomous practitioner who is well able to react intelligently and assertively with other health care professionals' (Robinson 1991). Apparently these writers see 'then and now' descriptions as convincing. But could it be true? Could the products of such a ritual-bound, task-orientated, inflexible past be the very people who would invent Project 2000? Perhaps its inventors were an élite few who somehow surmounted the ritualisms and clichés of their own archaic courses?

I find 'then and now' comparisons simplistic and in the context of the evolution of psychiatric nursing (Carpenter 1988; Nolan 1993) doubly so. History rarely proceeds in straight lines as Maben and Macleod Clark's own results show and there is even a sense in which the Project 2000 innovation has merely highlighted old problems or even made them worse.

Macleod Clark *et al.* (1996), however, are cautiously optimistic that Project 2000 students, 'even in the face of uncompromising ward routine, where the academic/clinical match cannot be perfect' will persevere safe in the knowledge that, ultimately, educational material which they currently see as irrelevant will have clinical application. This is a classical error of curriculum planners whose belief seems to be that life will follow whatever educational programmes they devise. There occurs a complete inability to recognise that concepts of education and training for practice should proceed from a consideration of the nature of patients' illnesses. Ryan (1989), for instance, suggests that Project 2000 is a kind of back-to-front approach wherein student nurses are given the extraordinary task of taking Project 2000 'thinking' into clinical placements some of which, as I have suggested, may be ill-disposed to accept it.

The ENB report

Sponsored by the English National Board for Nursing and Midwifery (ENB), Macleod Clark *et al.* (1996) closely analysed a wide range of issues pertaining to students, teachers and managers. The study was conducted in a context in which Project 2000 was seen as bringing radical change into British nurse education. Its opening chapter attempts to lay the foundation of what is seen as an inevitable outcome for nurse education, namely its proper place within the university system. In effect, a Whig history (Butterfield 1965) is presented whereby the past is construed as a battle between progressive and reactionary forces, with the progressives ultimately winning through. As Burke (1977) observes, what Butterfield meant by this was the tendency to overestimate similarities between past and present such as to fallaciously assume that people *intend* the consequences of their actions. Whereas, of course, the past can never sensibly will the present. For our purposes it is not enough to caution against the danger of doing this, as indeed Macleod Clark *et al.* do, but to point out that the construction of nursing history has often fallen prey to this fallacy and indeed until Brian Abel-Smith's (1960) *A History of the Nursing Profession* almost all nursing history was hagiographic as well as biased towards general nursing.

Inspection of the Macleod Clark *et al.* (1996) study bears out the Whig hypothesis. For example, they refer to a number of writers and historians who claimed that nurses desired some form of educational change (plausible) and that they sought this change in the form of a university- or academic-based system (not so plausible). As Menzies-Lyth (1988) acidly points out, 'the imposition of blueprints is simply further evidence of the desire to avoid the development of models from within and as an outcome of group processes which involve as many nurses as possible'. These are issues which ultimately professional historians will dissect. For the moment, I suggest that a reading of the nursing literature will reveal the concerns of a small number of highly motivated people (see Le Var 1997a, 1997b) occupying positions within nurse education and the higher echelons of nursing management. The majority of nurses however may be reluctant to enter abstract or lengthy debates about the nature of nursing. As several commentators have noted, theoretical and or ideological discussion has not been a major preoccupation of shop floor nurses (Caudill 1958; Davis 1981; White 1985).

In sickness and in health

Specifically, Macleod Clark *et al.* (1996: 107) speak of a shift from a sickness to a health model and much is made of this as both a necessary and appropriate development. However, the report also recognises that students perceive a lack of anatomy and physiology as well as knowledge about illnesses as a serious deficiency. In addition they also accept that most qualifiers take up their first post in a hospital. This is striking because having noted that Project 2000 was designed to 'address the changing needs of society in the twenty-first century, it is accepted that structures *are not yet in place* in the community for these goals to be realised' (my emphasis). Without overstating the case, even a cursory examination of community psychiatric care following the demise of the mental hospitals might have told them that. More generally, embarking upon educational courses on the basis of imagined, community-based, twenty-first century ills at a time when increasing numbers of people are ever more indebted to hospital and other medical technology is surprising.

Attributing weight

An important aspect of the Maben and Macleod Clark study was its interviews with students, teachers and managers involved with Project 2000 schemes. Overall, these interviews support the continuation of Project 2000 courses. However, whilst most of the interviewees were generally pleased, some of the managers worried about financial aspects of the new training and some students complained about a lack of support and organisation. Lack of organisation and planning seems to have been a fairly wide perception, something which is reflected in the anonymous letters which the *Nursing Times* (1997) received at the time. The main complaint of both managers and students, however, was that their courses lacked a proper emphasis on what they called basic nursing care. These criticisms notwithstanding, the report came to a favourable conclusion about the Project 2000 scheme overall. Complaints were attributed to 'teething problems', amenable to early amelioration.

Such optimism may have been misplaced however. For example, the deficiencies outlined by Maben and Macleod Clark are remarkably similar to other findings and bear a striking resemblance to those produced by students in response to my own inquiries. What seems to differ is the manner in which different researchers comprehend the criticisms. The bitterness which I have perceived behind student's responses to Project 2000 seems mysteriously absent in the reports of Macleod Clark *et al.* and others (Maben and Macleod Clark 1998; Elkan and Robinson 1995). My discussions with Project 2000 students across the country show that they are dismayed by the lack of preparation in clinical skills as well as what they see as an idiosyncratic exposure to sociological theory.

The Elkan and Robinson summary

In 1995 these writers reviewed nine studies which had evaluated various aspects of Project 2000. Essentially, they concluded that the Project 'had elicited overwhelming support'. Admittedly there were 'teething effects' but generally all was well and 'there could now be no question of turning the clock back' (Elkan and Robinson 1995: 391).

The teething effects were as follows:

1   The changes had been too rapidly introduced.
2   Students felt swamped by the breadth and disparate nature of the common foundation programme (CFP).
3   Lack of skills acquisition during the CFP.
4   The heavy emphasis during the CFP on Adult nursing.
5   Discrepancies between what is taught and actual clinical experience.
6   The CFP was too long.

Noticeably, most of these problems centred on the CFP and there was little disquiet coming from the branch programmes. Evidently, Elkan and Robinson were determined to look on the bright side. Apart from the 'no turning back' remark, they saw Project 2000 as having an inestimable value in providing high quality education with overwhelming support for the reforms and so forth. In fairness, they did advocate amending programmes in response to the various problems which they listed and time has indeed brought some changes in its wake. Common foundation programmes have been shortened in many institutes and more practical aspects are being incorporated into courses. However, the philosophical nature of the CFP, symbolising as it does those features believed to be unique to nursing as well as the place of nursing as a university-based discipline, remains unexamined. Whether the overwhelming support elicited by these writers is representative of the views of psychiatric nurses generally is not addressed by them.

These authors could hardly have been unaware of the depth of feeling which some psychiatric nurses had expressed towards CFP elements. One nursing director (McIntegart 1990) had complained of a loss of identity for psychiatric nursing yet according to Elkan and Robinson (1995: 389), his fears are borne out only to 'the very limited extent that the concept of a generic CFP has indeed been difficult to reconcile with the very different needs of students intending to undertake different branch programmes, particularly mental health branch students'.

It is worth quoting McIntegart's objection in full:

> The fear harboured for so long by psychiatric nurses that our unique role might be lost within a more generalised nurse model is now slowly becoming a reality. Project 2000 is the educational process that will squeeze the mental health nurse into a generalist mould. The nursing profession seems hell bent on creating an all-singing, all-dancing nurse, capable of anything and everything, and this could result in the demise of mental health nursing.
>
> (1990: 72)

Elkan and Robinson respond by labelling McIntegart's views as the product of 'a lobby' and they refuse to see it as an alternative perspective on nurse education. This kind of response is not unknown in nursing where intermittently there emerges a dominant ethos, model or orientation, highly favoured by the nursing establishment such that any objections to it are seen as 'troublemaking' or 'rocking the boat'. Evidence for the failure of such thinking, say Elkan and Robinson, is deduced by the fact that 'no one in the literature is advocating that mental health nurses leave nursing'. This is true but of little consequence unless you equate leaving Project 2000 as equivalent to leaving nursing.

The journal which published Elkan and Robinson's paper accepted a short response (Clarke 1996) in which I pointed to the fact that since Project 2000 had been trumpeted as major innovation, the assumption that nurse lecturers would be in a position to 'go against the grain' in criticising it seemed naïve. In my case my superior (now retired) had warned me to stop criticising the changes and that if I did not 'want to join in, there were plenty around who did'. Indeed, the general period of Project 2000 implementation from the early 1980s onwards corresponds to that period in industrial relations in which there appeared to exist a corporate 'climate of fear'. This was the period of the introduction of short-term contracts and it seemed to be asking a lot of people that they criticise the activities of their respective organisations whilst at the same time trying to secure mortgages on fixed-term employment contracts.

My view is that a self-congratulatory element accompanied not only the change itself but in addition much of the review material which followed. The context of these reviews is that some are funded by the English National Board (ENB) which is a constituent body of the organisation (UKCC) which implemented the changes in the first place. Indeed in some cases evaluations of Project 2000 effectiveness have been carried out by people whose responsibility it is to deliver Project 2000 courses to literally hundreds of students.

Degrees of influence

Following its implementation, evidence of the success of Project 2000 quickly turned into a rush for an all-graduate teaching staff. As one respondent said, 'it was a case of getting a degree, any degree' (Kirk *et al.* 1997: 1039). A tendency to respond with alacrity when faced with new proposals is a common event in nursing. The Robbins Committee on Higher Education, as long ago as 1963, commented on the nursing profession's proclivity to 'uncritically accept knowledge', their appreciation of anything new or innovative as 'received wisdom' coupled with a tendency to implement changes quickly. Elkan and Robinson (1995) refer to a subject of Payne *et al.* (1991) who said that the implementation of Project 2000 was like 'laying railway lines as the train is arriving' and Le Var (1997a, 1997b) reported that the UKCC had shortened the original two-year time scale for the project to eighteen months. Obviously some pressure existed to push these changes through fairly quickly.

Who is it for?

Menzies-Lyth (1988) saw Project 2000 as representing little more than the imposition of a grand scheme clearly regarded by some as an important development but with questionable evidence that the broad mass of British nurses wanted it. Le Var's statement that 'wide consultation ensured that the resultant policy did not represent only the views of the power structure' does not fit with the shortened 'consultation period' which she also reported. Le Var, an officer of the ENB, also speaks of the contributions 'behind the scenes' of key players 'in the profession', contributions, she says, *'likely to have been vital'* (my emphasis). I doubt that the rank and file were consulted very much at all. My recollection is of Project 2000 literature being distributed to hospital wards but without any attempt to canvass views in any systematic form.

As matters stand there appears to be emerging some disquiet from the Department of Health as to the continuing viability of university-based nurse education (Phillips 1999). More specifically there is now some acknowledgement that psychiatric nursing has been compromised by the common foundation elements of Project 2000 programmes. As the Mental Health Nursing Review Team (1994) conceded, it is probably too early to go back and it is true that the constant changes of recent years makes the thought of further change unbearable. Having said that, there are important questions which psychiatric nurses need to address. For example, what is the nature of mental illness and how should nurses respond to it? What role should users have in evaluating psychiatric nursing interventions? How do we address the political elements which attend care in the community for psychiatric patients? What is the responsibility of psychiatric nurses in respect of policing community-based patients? How can psychiatric nurses resolve these issues when caught up in an educational curriculum which has to take account of the needs of prospective medical surgical nurses, a curriculum which contains no recognition of psychiatric nursing as a qualitatively different exercise to other forms of nursing?

What is required is an independent psychiatric curriculum with direct entry for applicants. To a lesser extent what is also needed is an independent national centre for psychiatric nursing studies. Such a unit, licensed by parliament, would promote the welfare of professional nurses as well as health service users. In addition to the usual activities of audit and validation it would also serve to define psychiatric nursing as a unique social activity.

10 The search for conclusions

It was Desmond Cormack (1983) who observed that most nurse writing was prescriptive and whilst he was referring mainly to British nurses, recent American writing has been just as prescriptive, indeed more so. In their ceaseless quest to formulate a unique nursing knowledge, American theorists have yielded to artificial concepts, a proliferation of nursing models and processes being the main result. Not that the influence of these theorists is limited to America. They have had a significant influence in Britain especially amongst educationalists, curriculum developers and professional spokespersons generally. As we finalise our analysis therefore, we do so from the vantage point of the prescriptive nature of nursing ideas, the proclamation of these ideas by élitist groups and the possibility that the broad mass of nurses may actually be committed to more practical conceptions of the nature of their work.

Relatives and professionals

According to Schlotfeldt (1996: 101) 'Nursing has been in existence for almost one and a half centuries'. This statement negatively defines that which preceded Nightingale as 'not nursing'. The irony is that had the Lady with the Lamp had her way, nursing would still be an amateur event (Nightingale 1952) with much of it delivered by patients' relatives or vocational caregivers. The latter point provokes a consideration of medicine as a conjoint, preventative activity shared between clinicians and public. Recent manifestations of this have been the transfer of prescriptive medicines onto the free market as well as an added emphasis on information given to patients both by professionals but also via self-help groups, user movements and the mass media. Equally, the advent of community care (DoH 1990) leaves many patients in the care of relatives.

What these developments represent is a formal recognition of the role of relatives and interested others in the care of sick people. Of course there is nothing new in this. Sick people have always been cared for by female relatives and only in unusual instances were they removed to hospitals (Porter 1996). However, from the nineteenth century until the middle of the twentieth, hospitals began to cater more and more for a variety of ills; from psychiatric to infectious disorders, from chronic ills to care of the dying (McKeown and Lowe 1974). Given that general hospitals now concentrate on curing illnesses and with lengthy stays following treatment being frowned upon, and given that psychiatric hospitals are now seen as somewhat undesirable, we may ask what differences exist between nursing carried out by relatives or volunteers as opposed to professionals? Brecher (1988) states that a professional's respect for his patient 'is not just that respect which one human being owes another' for, if it was, 'there would be no difference between the carer's obligation to the patient and general moral obligation'. This suggests that relationships with one's loved-ones are part of such a general obligation whereas the professional relationship is more circumscribed. However the distinction is not always obvious. For instance, Watson (1989) argues that even when caring for strangers, they (the strangers) are never completely anonymous. We know that strangers are human for example and moreover, all of us share in a moral obligation to the society of humanity as a whole. The practical side of this obligation is seen in the fact that few of us have not nursed a relative or friend at some stage in our lives.

Yet, as a professional activity, nursing would seem to require more than a general moral obligation by which to define itself, some other yardstick by which to separate itself from the amateur. Without excluding universal obligations, many nurses would say that their knowledge base is what outstrips the lay nursing activist. It is knowledge which supports their status as expert practitioners. Responding to recent criticisms of Project 2000, Sue Studdy, Dean of City University Nursing School, London, stated:

> Nurses are expected to have a wide range of knowledge so they can undertake evidence based practice.
>
> (1999: 8)

Nursing expertise

People enter professional relationships when they believe that their wants can be met in ways that cannot be met elsewhere. Hence they consult doctors, lawyers, architects and so on. It is not clear if this kind of professional construct encompasses counselling, nursing, teaching or social work. In respect of social workers for instance, British legislators, when framing the Mental Health Act (1959), defined their role as little different to that of patients' relatives in the implementation of detention orders. In addition to how their role is defined by legislation, nurses have also defined their task from a humanistic, holistic perspective. Is it possible from within such a perspective for them to lay claim to professional status? Can they, like doctors, architects and lawyers, proclaim a defined expertise in the service of others? Or is nursing a vaguer, more broad-based undertaking, an expression of humanitarianism, a basic instinct to care?

Basic nursing care

Setting to one side technical jobs like changing drips and inserting catheters, most practising nurses probably engage in what is called basic nursing care. For instance, an incapacitated patient needs lots of this kind of care and we can reasonably ask what special knowledge underpins its delivery. After all, lay persons deliver such care as effectively as anyone, for instance the primary carers of young infants. In respect of technical tasks, many people are routinely involved in resuscitation, first aid, giving injections and so on and it appears that these can be administered with minimal supportive knowledge.

However, if the knowledge which is claimed to differentiate professionals from their lay counterparts is of the kind which does underpin such tasks, then some nurses do indeed appear to want more of it, presumably to increase the effectiveness of their interventions. However the question is whether the possession of this technical knowledge differentiates nurses as a profession. The answer to that depends on the extent to which the nurses' technical interventions constitute nursing. In my view they do not.

Of course, nurses must acquire knowledge and skills so as to carry out their nursing successfully whilst affording themselves an informed view about medical matters. However, at what level of knowledge acquisition would they be satisfied? How close to the knowledge levels of medics for example would such learning have to be? Would there occur a point at which it would come to resemble the knowledge levels of medics, and on hitting that plateau, would it not make sense to exchange the title 'nurse' for 'doctor'? Specifically, how detailed a knowledge of circulatory systems is required to nurse coronary patients? Is it the same as that needed to treat them? The question is resolutely problematic because experienced nurses may be more *competent* than junior doctors whose knowledge is presumably greater but at this stage of their careers chiefly academic. The nursing knowledge, in these instances, is comprised of clinical experience and the kinds of 'on the job' competencies which are often a product of custom and practice.

Nurse, would you mind …

That these competencies are recognised in the work place is evidenced by nurses being requested by surgeons (typically it seems) to perform minor surgical procedures (*Nursing Times* 1995). *Towards Tomorrow* (BMA 1996) actually requests that nurses re-arrange their roles so as to take on what were formerly medical tasks. Overall, the nursing response to such requests has been ambivalent. Certainly, occupational domains shift over time and a re-evaluation of the relative responsibilities of doctors and nurses may be overdue. Currently, we may be seeing the emergence of a medicarer with basic nursing care being cost-driven on the backs of vocationally trained nurses. Because these vocational nurses are freed from the responsibility of diagnosing and prescribing they are enabled to deal with the effects of prescriptions and treatments on patients thus fulfilling the traditional view of nursing care. However, where this leaves the professional nurse with her new knowledge base is hard to say.

Clearly, nursing knowledge which derives from a biologically based curriculum cannot compete with medicine. Something else is obviously needed if nursing is to achieve a different identity. It cannot base its identity on medical interventions such as performing catheterisations since the knowledge which governs such interventions stems from medical sciences. This explains the attractiveness of humanistic models and especially holism as an alternative route towards professional identity. However, common sense entails that any movement towards separateness by nurses is going to have to come to terms with the inevitable closeness of occupational co-dependency of nurses and doctors and where the medical status of patients is crucial.

In psychiatric practice, alternatively, the nature of what constitutes illness is so genuinely problematic that attempts to legitimise its medical basis are fairly common. These attempts typically comprise an exposition of the physiological basis of mental illness coupled with an invalidation of interpersonal relationships with patients. Interestingly, it is this interpersonal approach which is welcomed by psychiatric users as opposed to so-called objective psychiatry (Campbell 1995). Although the conditions of psychiatric practice leave open the possibility of alternative concepts of psychiatric distress, psychiatric nurses have also preferred a close liaison with their medical colleagues. As general nurses espouse a holistic framework whilst carrying out their medical duties, so do psychiatric nurses – the majority of whom continue to work in institutional settings (Brooker and White 1998) – continue to dispense drugs whilst declaring their allegiance to person-centred care. This is not to say that a person-centred approach would not contribute to the well-being of patients in medical, surgical or psychiatric settings. However, as Salvage (1985) observes, whilst patients do indeed judge the quality of their relationships with nurses along an emotional continuum, they by no means seek the warm and empathic relationships which some nurse-counsellors imagine. In this respect, Bjork (1995) has shown that medical patients consistently demonstrate a high regard for nurses' attention to hygiene and comfort as well as their contribution to medical treatments. This suggests that the holistic concerns of contemporary nurses are not necessarily shared by patients or even by many practising nurses who, says Sharma (1992), continue to attach importance to the biophysical aspects of their job.

Yet a number of post-Project 2000 complaints about the lack of basic nursing have been made by doctors (Harris 1995), students (Williamson 1998) and the general public (Peters 1995; Phillips 1999). These views do not seem to tally with the 'caring profession' rhetoric of recent years. Neither, however, do they reflect my contention that the majority of practising nurses continue to carry out medically prescribed treatments and associated nursing. Yet such complaints have proliferated particularly since the implementation of Project 2000 courses.

My belief is that complaints about basic care are anecdotal, the outcome of observations of simple bad practice and related to Project 2000 only inasmuch as they reflect the prejudices of those who oppose the notion of professionalised nursing full stop. It is true that since the inception of Project 2000, older systems of care delivery and the disciplinary structures which monitored them have fallen by the wayside. Contemporary nursing is more committed to the idea of the individual as a psycho-social entity and this may mean in some circumstances a loss of the standards of hygienic excellence and physical care which went hand in hand with routinised nursing. The truth is, that nursing has reached a point where it no longer has much of a coherent sense of its own worth or even in some cases identity. The nursing base is undecided because confused. If it takes its lead from a medical model then this hardly counts as nursing, more a kind of assistant doctoring. If it subscribes to holistic principles, then this poses serious problems in terms of what can be eliminated from traditional practice. In psychiatric nursing, any change involving a shift away from medicine would necessarily involve redefining the nature of mental illness.

Convergence on caring

A constant feature of debates about the nature of nursing is the concept of care (Barker *et al.* 1995). Of course, if caring for people is about serving their needs, then it may be possible to do this without caring; The nurse who manages her ward with hygienic precision might *appear* not to care, preoccupied with routine she might frown upon talking to patients but her patients might nevertheless be well cared for in many respects. Further, some nurses, perhaps through frustration, might hate their patients – rather in the way that one could strangle one's crying child – or their job, yet perform their responsibilities conscientiously and fairly. After all, caring *for* someone is not the same as caring about them. An example of this might be the positive regard shown to paedophiles by nurses who privately harbour disgust towards them (Clarke 1991). In this instance, nurses act from duty in keeping with their sense of professionalism. To what extent this reflects an element of deception is debatable as is the willingness of the recipient to be so deceived.

In general, nursing is a largely humanitarian effort where the nursing performance may reflect life experiences as much as the acquisition of academic knowledge. This is important because professions are defined largely by the nature of their knowledge base (Walby *et al.* 1994). As such, we can agree that skills such as resuscitation and first aid are essential to nursing but also that many groups in society possess these. Nurses should equip themselves with those skills of course, and they have. However, it is when they aspire towards more abstract areas that problems occur. Some have criticised the appropriation of excess theoretical baggage as unnecessary. For example both Allen (1990) and Williamson (1998) objected to the concentrated diet of social science, delivered literally miles from clinical areas, which they felt threatened the credibility of their nurse training. Their view was that nurses ought to be more concerned with issues relevant to basic practice.

Currently however, the educationalist's idea of a knowledgeable doer requires an academic grounding and the prevailing tendency is to generate theory which transcends patients' physical needs and the care which would normally attend them. Another dimension of this, as Kitson (1996: 313) notes, is that 'an élitist nursing agenda' has been nudged towards 'an advanced nursing practice reform with nurse leaders effectively alienating the majority of nurses who give care'. What Kitson describes is a cleavage between a university as opposed to a vocational approach. Whilst the question of what constitutes an educational base for the former has to some extent been answered what remains unclear is how much of an educational base such vocational training should have. Kitson regards vocation, especially its allusions to 'the nurse as angel, harlot, mother-figure, battle axe', with suspicion. However, this neglects the historical validity of these terms as well as the way in which their use by other parties (doctors, administrators) has worked to inhibit the development of nurses as a gender-specific group. The point is, whatever the education of the vocational nurse, logic entails that it will be less than for university nurses and that it is this which will separate the two groups. However, it hardly follows that university-educated nurses would have less of a caring capacity than their more practical colleagues. For if the vocational ethic implies an imperative to care, and I believe it does, it seems to me that this ought not to prohibit a university education. The question then is, should vocationally motivated students receive additional academic input and if they should, what would its nature be? In recent years, its nature has been heavily influenced by humanistic thinking and the kind of holistic philosophising which underpins counselling psychology. Kitson regards this as some kind of betrayal with nurses 'selling their caring birthright for a mess of psychological pottage' (1996: 313). However, working out what that birthright is remains a problem.

In general, it is hardly surprising that nurses have opted for humanistic principles since the fuzzy nature of these principles defies precise description and so resembles the caring role which as yet is also unspecified. There is a certain effrontery in nurses pretending to have an edge on caring, and to assert, as some of them do, that caring is some kind of birthright is silly particularly if the idea that 'nursing is caring' amounts to little more than a tautology. A reliance on caring as some kind of philosophical wellspring only leads back to vocation. If this is not enough, if nurses seek a university-level knowledge base, then either they settle for the 'psychological pottage' of counselling responses, build up a repertoire of secondary medical skills or settle instead for some kind of scientific basis for the meaning of caring. But in what sense, actually, *could* caring be scientific? I will address this question later but first I want to look further at the idea of nursing as a wider social activity.

A basic rethink

A basic rethink is needed involving notions of responsibility of individuals in a society to each other, relationships of members of families to the larger community and the nature of the relationship of professionals to those being served. This would constitute a starting point for an examination of nursing issues which may possess a medical component but which cannot be detached from wider social considerations. In his book *Taking Care* (1987) David Smail pleads for a sense of community responsibility in dealing with people's welfare. Smail's view is that many human problems previously seen as coming from individualised pathology can be helped by removing or adjusting socially inhibiting factors.

However, it is uncommon for psychiatric nurses to give much consideration to social and political systems as causal mechanisms of mental disorder. Not that nursing lacks a political dimension. Over the years both Jane Salvage (1985) and Rosemary White (1985) have argued for such a dimension in nursing practice and Salvage's current editorship of the *Nursing Times* has produced a 'mission statement' which aims to be both 'radical' and 'challenging'. However, practising nurses rarely define their work in political or even social terms and community psychiatric nurses, perhaps surprisingly, have been peculiarly unable to achieve more than a moderate articulation of the growing social desperation of hospital discharged and socially bereft client groups. With few exceptions, the community psychiatric nursing literature reveals the apolitical (even conservative) stance endemic to British psychiatry (see *Community Psychiatric Nursing Journal* for the period 1984–94). There even occurs an open declaration of ideological neutrality: witness Carr's (1984) claim that the anti-psychiatric activities of some community psychiatric nurses was 'a case of pragmatism rather than a counter-ideology changing with established patterns of practice'. The current emphasis on 'serious and enduring' mental illness (Brooker and Repper 1998) is similarly less an expression of a concern about the social and economic neglect of patients and more an ideological statement about the physical nature of mental illness. Indeed in *Serious Mental Health Problems in the Community* (Brooker and Repper 1998) neither author was able to say what was meant by serious mental illness in what purported to be a major text on the topic.

How nurses are seen

To a degree, nurses have been hemmed in by society's view of them. Societal views of course depend upon which segment of society is canvassed but by and large the nursing image has been one of selfless devotion and unyielding dedication to the sick. It is a picture often summarised by the word 'caring' although as we are beginning to see, vocational concepts of nursing – and the suggestion here is that caring is difficult to define *because* of its vocational dimension – can bring trouble in their wake.

To begin with, caring in nursing presupposes a given set of characteristics which go a long way towards determining what a nurse is. These characteristics are virtuous dispositions to fortitude, compassion and so on and they form a powerful conative element in the life of the nurse. In other words the vocational element stems not from profession but is an example of one's values. It implies an acquisition of knowledge, but knowledge which will be secondary to establishing an atmosphere conducive to well-being, healing and recovery; hence, you might say, nursing ethics. However, as Smail indicates, caring is not some kind of internal faculty possessed by nurses or anyone else. It is not some skill, some emotional gift or learnt acquisition. Rather is it a phenomenon which stretches beyond the individual and into the experiences of those to whom it is directed. It is relational, communal and essentially undefinable.

For Brown, Kitson and McKnight (1992), the professionalising of nursing into a skills-based problem-centred activity misses the central point about learning experientially to care for others. Irrespective of the situation in general nursing, prior to the commencement of Project 2000, such experiential learning had been a defining characteristic of psychiatric nurse education. Now that this is lost (for the moment anyway) it becomes possible to see nursing skills as merely another 'professionalising up' of universal human responses. Perversely, this diminishes the responses it seeks to elevate by interposing a conceptual framework between them and any honest reaction to them by patients or other involved parties. Hunt (1994) suggests that this conceptualising is but another expression of the nursing belief that there is always a right way to do things and he identifies the teaching of communication skills as an example of this. Likewise, Gournay (1995) currently seeks a transformation of mental nursing from humanist carers into medical proselytes in search of the 'right' (enduring and serious) patients to 'nurse'. In either case the idea of nursing as a basic human response is abolished and replaced in both cases by professionalised responses of precarious quality.

There *is* a noble element in nursing, of course: only good comes from self-scrutiny and the will to do better. But self-regard too easily slides into the desire to *be* better. Contemporary nursing curricula fail to apprehend those features which represent the vocation of nursing (Williams 1978), the heart of which is a disposition to virtue, a virtue which values events *between* people (and within societies) and whose devotion to compassion and tenderness enriches our culture. Extravagant curricula and parodies of medical knowledge and ethics interferes with the quality of being with someone who is ill. Even the act of listening has given way to battalions of counselling poseurs with their ridiculous theories of living (such as transactional analysis) and absurd admonitions such as: 'Yes but what I *really* hear you say', within a nursing framework which, increasingly, has the look of nursing by appointment written all over it.

Williams (1978) observes that it is a patient's helplessness which lies at the centre of those tasks which embody the image of 'the nurse' and that this verifies the traditional identity of nursing from both the nurses' and the publics' point of view. She asserts that it is through service in a hospital that people are admitted to the title of nurse and that nursing is still predominantly about dealing with illness in a hands-on way and irrespective of any conceptual sophistry which may attend such care. Psychiatric nursing surveys (Brooker and White 1998) reinforce this position as do the ongoing crises concerning nursing shortages in the National Health Service, crises which are entirely to do with the provision of hospital care.

Having said this, too much emphasis on hospitalisation or the service ethic of nursing can result in a skewed picture. Quoting from Greer (1973), Benner (1984) imbues nurses with 'compassion, empathy, innocence and sensuality' and, apparently, identifies these qualities as uniquely female. This seems an idealisation of sorts and it is problematic mainly because of the way it characterises the nursing relationship as a human response. Elements of loving relationships incorporated into professional settings can be risky and one suspects that the creation of codes of conduct partly seeks to curb the imagined consequences which such intimacies can bring. Brecher (1995) suggests that if you make a practice of what is in ordinary circumstances an act of friendship (helping a friend who has flu for instance) then you may need, for both parties, a code for that which does not in friendship need governance. Inevitably, it becomes a problem of weighing up the transformation involved in nursing strangers as opposed to relatives and friends. For example, is it possible to confront human pain, over and over, as if it were that of a loved one? As stated, whilst the impulse to care is a vocational attribute, it requires some degree of impersonal structure in its different situations of care. For if intimacy can personify tenderness, equally can it spawn violence, something born out by the extraordinary number of abuses (Robb 1967; DHSS 1969, 1971, 1972, 1974; Stockwell 1972; Lunder 1987; Blom-Cooper 1992; Vernon 1995) which occur in our hospitals as well as individual outrages (against children, for instance). In addition, it might be the case that befriended patients would be unable to voice those needs and demands which they might do within less personal relationships. Introducing the personal into professional nursing may deepen the patient's responsibilities to the nurse and that might not always be a good thing. That it occurs in families is irrelevant since we are not the patient's family. As such, should we not avoid burdening people with superfluous friendships, especially at times of letting go? Alternatively, is not one of the justifications for professional nursing the alleviation of unbearable stress which is an accompaniment of nursing relatives? For instance the situation of a forty-year-old woman having to address the infantile needs of an eighty-year-old parent and everything that this entails both physically and psychologically.

Objective, subjective

According to Alison Kitson:

> The nursing profession is split between its poorly understood and poorly articulated commitment to care and its more strident resolve to provide individualised deliberative patient care – designed to promote recovery.
>
> (1988: 24)

It is Kitson's view that nurses emulate the medical profession in their desire to evolve frameworks which have a look of objectivity about them. However, in embracing an objective science, says Kitson, nurses have neglected the sensual or subjective elements of what they do. Kitson feels that having opted for rationalism, a debate about caring cannot proceed since the subjective element has been thrown out. Caring, she says, is simply not an objective process and whilst few would disagree with that, difficulties begin once you try to apprehend what this subjective element is.

The problem, it seems to me, is the sheer impossibility of capturing the essence of 'this indefinable care' (McFarlane 1988: 19), an impossibility which has led to intense preoccupation with the artificiality of conceptual models and processes. In effect, these models represent little more than what one might call 'aspirational knowledge'. In one obvious sense, this relates to occupational advancement whereas in another, it attempts to define reality through discourse. This sets up contradictions since discourse is always one step ahead of reality. That being the case, one must inquire which discourses operate within which realities or, to put it differently, whose interests are best served by different professional discourses. The point being that power and influence have little to do with knowledge *per se* but a lot to do with how medical language constructs and mediates professional settings. For example the nurse might have a Ph.D. in microbiology but it is the doctor who is legitimised by society to direct patients' treatment and, until now at any rate, accorded the right to do this without contradiction in principle. In part, it is the sheer intractability of the medical hegemony which has forced nurses to construct alternative perceptions of care, conceptions involving additions to the physical, the carving out of some caring domain over and above medical ways of seeing things.

However, because the premises by which this is done are often vague and rhetorical it becomes difficult to disentangle what is intended or what the consequences for care might be. For example, observe the complicated way in which Holden writes about propositional knowledge:

As an art, nursing rests on the delicate interplay between propositional knowledge and nonpropositional knowledge associated with the mastery of psychomotor skills. As a science, nursing draws heavily on propositional scientific knowledge that is then applied in the practice area. But most important, it is the expert nurses, with their impressive reservoir of nonarticulated, perceptual propositional knowledge who transport nursing from a humdrum world of honest toil to the scientific realm of creative caring.

(1996: 33)

Holden typifies the soaring heights school of nursing philosophy. At face value this looks like a very impressive statement. Close inspection however reveals a series of illogical connections and unspecified terms. What, for instance, is 'nonarticulated, perceptual propositional knowledge'? What does the 'scientific realm of creative caring' mean? How can propositions be 'not articulated'? If the answer (cf. Dawkins 1998, chapter 8) is that they are 'special kinds of propositions which lie within perceptual fields' then my guess is that perceptual psychologists would find this ridiculous (see Gregory 1997) given that perception is an active process anyway.

Deeper into philosophy

Deciphering the conceptual basis of nursing is a minefield of 'shoulds', 'musts' and 'oughts'. Consider the following from Parse (1992) (quoted by Davies and Lynch 1995: 30): 'The human lives at multidimensional realms of the universe all at once, freely choosing ways of becoming as meaning is given in situations.'

One barely apprehends the possible meanings within this sentence. Suspecting as much, Davies and Lynch (1995: 390) comment that 'each person will make meaning of the concept of caring within the spectrum of their own reality and such a construct further magnifies the pluri-dimensional complexity of caring'. I quote these authors because they are good examples of the inscrutable syntax used by recent nursing scholars, endless epistles of neologisms, metaphors, *non-sequiturs* and funny combinations, all designed to hide the fact that what is being discussed is the straightforward question of caring for others in a manner which embraces the basic decencies of everyday life. The latter identifies caring as a compassionate response however and this is objected to by the scholars because it re-invokes the poisoned chalice of nursing as a vocation. For nurse philosophers, it is not enough just to care, one's caring must be transformed from a human condition response into something which represents the actions of a professional group. What these nursing scholars seek therefore is the added on bit, the extra dimension which qualifies nursing as a uniquely new and different (to medicine) function. Yet, what they invariably seem to produce are complex models whose chief characteristics are density and a built-in resistance to anything that resembles actual living. It may seem an unfair comparison but one immediately thinks of modern couturiers designing clothes so outlandish as to be practicably unwearable but which are trundled down the catwalk nevertheless.

Thus the proliferation of mannered pronouncements, tortured descriptions and circuitous writing all topped off with the admission that tight definitions are difficult because of the elusiveness of caring. As Felicity Stockwell (1985: 11) says: 'It is extremely difficult to find words to make adequate sense of nursing.' I would say that it is as mindless an exercise as trying to define love. Notice, in particular, the proliferation of secondary terms, that nursing is knowledgeable doing, or purposive, or deliberative (Orlando 1961) or that it is a tapestry (Arendt 1992). One encounters this verbal sleight of hand again and again. Johnson (1996: 49), for instance, has a version which she calls artful nursing, a version which requires *habitus*. *Habitus*, says Johnson, is 'a stable disposition to act in a certain way that is acquired via exercise and use'. It is not enough to have theoretical knowledge, she says, so much as to own it in a way which allows one to proceed in a spontaneous, intuitive, caring manner.

As Davies and Lynch (1995) acknowledge, such confusion is hardly surprising given the 'immense diversity in definitions and conceptualisations of caring'. Having fine-combed the literature on caring, Sourial's (1997: 1191) conclusion, derived from Walker and Advant (1995), was that even when analyses of caring are rigorous and precise the 'end product will differ from person to person and therefore it is always a tentative result'.

The fact is, scholarship has done little to identify caring as a concept. However, why should it have done when it would be as easy to reconceptualise love, respect, cruelty, faith or hate? Such obstacles have proved to be no barrier, however, so that ever upwards and onwards nurse theorists reach for the transpersonal as one more pathway to final truth.

Tackling this question head on

On what grounds *exactly* could a nurse not implement a medical prescription? Given that medical training confers authority to determine treatments, in what circumstances could such treatments be modified by nurses? Insofar as the medical authority derives from a basis in reason (May 1993), that is, the accumulation of years of trial and error reasoning which all states validate by statute, how therefore can a position derived from humanistic principles hope to entertain equal credibility in situations where people's medical and surgical illnesses are central? Of course, medical authority extends no further than this and one would hardly accept a doctor's ruling on financial or legal matters for instance. Equally, nurses are obliged to intervene if physicians act either intentionally or mistakenly to harm patients.

De Raeve (1993) raises the issue of nurses' prescribing as an area of blurred responsibilities between doctors and nurses. The doctor's authority is limited, she says, by a growing prescriptive expertise of nurses which, by definition, suggests a diminishing obligation to defer to that authority. There is something in this because if nurses were to acquire more and more medical knowledge, to perform more and more medical tasks, then they would eventually reach level pegging with the medics. However, who then would do the nursing? This is the problem with de Raeve's position which is that nurse prescribing is not nursing and granted that such prescribing becomes commonplace, it must also be seen in a context of the deregulation of medicines generally such that anyone can now buy, in high street chemists, medicines which were prescriptive only a short while ago.

The mental health dimension

Discussions about power, authority and conduct become more problematic in the context of psychiatric practice. Here, illness categories are by no means as clear cut as in physical medicine. According to Davidson (1998), nurses lack a defined role in relation to mental illness lacking as they do a prestigious level in the psychiatric hierarchy. This results in a reliance on medical thinking so as to account for their position both theoretically and administratively. Davidson represents a school of thought (see also Barker and Davidson 1998) which seeks to enhance the nursing role in respect of enabling patients to 'tell their story'. Emphasising the client's narrative, they say, leads to demystification of psychiatric distress and an empowerment of clients. As Barker and Davidson insist:

> If we choose to move from the medical view we so often rely on, there is certainly no reason why we should be any less proficient in the dispensation of comfort and in the supply of this co-presence than those who have trained as doctors, psychotherapists or other more highly valued professionals.
>
> (1998: 63)

Part of the problem with this approach, and something which Gournay (1995) and others make much of, is that it leans heavily on literary, somewhat digressive, discourses which simply defy measurement or control. An example of such discourse is Barker and Davidson's (1998) distinction between the psychiatric and mental health nurse. Whereas, they say, the psychiatric nurse identifies a client's problems, mental health nurses facilitate the day-to-day experiences of individuals as they 'proceed down their life path'. In effect, they say, the psychiatric nurse, like the psychiatrist, makes a pretence at ideological neutrality, generally disregarding ethical and political elements which mediate mental illness. Whereas the mental health nurse operates along a wider, ethically influenced front, psychiatric nurses continue their timeless role of assisting doctors in the medicalisation of social problems whilst keeping faith that one day all will be biochemically revealed. In this analysis,

psychiatric nursing prides itself on having shrugged off subjective philosophising in favour of a more empirical view. However, that mental health is
objective in the sense of being more than an expression of the values of
psychiatry or the cultural norms of a society is dubious. That mental illness
is no less objective than, and analogous to, physical illness is just not true.
What happens in practice, however, is that this (hypothetically) diagnosable
mental illness is used to account for certain socially disruptive behaviours
which would otherwise be seen as morally or socially reprehensible. In effect,
one responds to these social disruptions not in any moral sense (of, let's say,
outrage) but in an objective, humane, way which defines them as illnesses
and so allows them to be treated. Obviously, conflict may arise if morality
runs counter to psychiatric practice, especially where forced detention, seclu-
sion and physical treatments are an issue. Most psychiatric nurses appear
untroubled by their long association with these processes and only rarely
acknowledge their custodial role. When it is acknowledged, it is usually
dressed in the finery of this or that euphemism, be it challenging behaviour
units, forensic nursing and so on. Intuitively, mental illness invites a wider
consideration of the lives of affected individuals. If dealing with someone's
psychological distress at the level of illness denies the question of how illness
is experienced, how much more invalid are responses which require incarcer-
ation as a necessary prerequisite to treatment.

The psychologically minded nurse

Having said that, if psychiatric nurses eschew biological approaches and opt
instead for psychological strategies then they adopt the mantle of mental
health and proceed to operate in a relatively non-medical way. If one then
asks them what they do they might respond: 'transactional analysis', 'gestalt
therapy', 'behaviour therapy' or a range of other psychological therapies.
One might then inquire precisely how these count as nursing. For example, if
one looked into two therapy rooms and saw, in one, a clinical psychologist
treat a patient using cognitive-behaviour therapy and, in another, a nurse do
the same, by what rule could you distinguish one as nursing? There appears
to be no satisfactory answer to this other than to call them both nursing. But
this is not right since it absurdly leaves open the question of what nursing is!
Of course, some may consider philosophical inquiries into the nature of
nursing as idiosyncratic. Ought nurses not content themselves with legal and
dictionary definitions? According to Diels (1994: 120): 'Nursing does not
defy definition, it is simply so huge that it cannot be distilled satisfactorily
into one or two pithy sentences.'

In other words, it does defy definition because pithy sentences are what
definitions are about. Part of the difficulty is an inability to be precise about
that area of care for which one actually has exclusive responsibility. In other
words, it is not alone what nurses do which matters (they do a great deal) but
on whose authority they do it. According to Diels (1994: 120), whether nurses

wish to take on new functions 'is not an issue of definition; it is an issue of control, including economic control, for if something must be done "under supervision", then it cannot be billed separately. And guess who collects the dough.' By 'supervision', of course, Diels means the medical profession.

For Kitson (1997), the viability of the nursing profession is about the accumulation of knowledge and a degree of control within the workplace. As such, evaluating nursing contributions is difficult given nursing's relative youth and the fact that both its knowledge and practice is mediated by the practice of medicine. Whilst there has been some shift in nurse–doctor relationships psychiatric nurses continue to express feelings of dis-empowerment at a time when they are being asked to empower others. The further paradox is that such empowerment must go hand-in-hand with a Government National Service Framework which requires psychiatric nurses to adopt a policing role in respect of patients seen as potentially dangerous or anti-social. For all of their claims to autonomous practitioner status, there is a sense in which community psychiatric nurses are being required to take on a role they would hardly assume for themselves. Yet again, they seem at the beck and call of an overriding medical ideology (enshrined in law) which shows little hesitation in locking patients up so as to treat them. Whereas clinical judgement was once about care and treatment we can see that it has now assumed a more sinister quality of controlling those who might pose a threat to the community. Yet again does psychiatry respond to the challenge of managing the risk to society, reconstructing itself as a thin white line between normalcy and the imagined consequences of not policing the mad.

Yet more euphemisms

What one seeks is an ethical and legal governance for the application of science in human affairs. This would entail merging the scientific process and caring into something new. The pursuance of science may well be motivated by care. One might also have a sense of care in science in the sense of precision. However, the notion of caring *as* science seems problematic. Kitson (1996) makes the attempt with what she calls 'skilled companionship' where the science element is the skill aspect whilst the companionship element falls between two stools of intimacy and distance. Companionship is described thus:

> There is a closeness that is not sexually stereotyped; it implies movement and change and requires commitment and mutuality. The skills of companionship are in being able to sense the need of the other person and accommodate oneself to the other's idiosyncrasies, to help the person onward by enabling them to see how the journey can be accomplished,

and to guard against the imposition of routines which make the patient feel trapped.

(1996: 1650)

One need not even substitute client for patient to see the similarities between this and much of Carl Rogers' writing: it neither adds to concepts of empathy, acceptance, being with etc. any more than it detracts from them. Actually, as recently as 1980, Rogers had stated that empathy means: 'Frequently checking with him/her as to the accuracy of your sensings, and being guided by the responses you receive. You are a confident companion to the person in his/her inner world' (Rogers 1980: 142).

It is just such a humanistic approach which Barker *et al.* (1998) utilise in opposition to growing positivism in health care and they further assert that their interpersonal approach is as 'eminently testable' as any other. However, by testing they would agree that this would be by qualitative methods and this raises a difficulty for the advocates of positivism since they fundamentally reject the premises upon which subjective research is based. Certainly, there appears little more we can do with the issue of what constitutes relationships or why they matter.

For Ritter (1997) it is time to stop pseudo-philosophising and instead do whatever gets nurses up the league table of the Research Assessment Exercise where owning up to the correctness of medical diagnosis and its treatment by medical/cognitive methods would seem to be a starting point. There is a strong pragmatism at work here, a belief that interventions which can be shown to work with seriously ill patients are the only ones worthy of attention. Nurses who reject this viewpoint probably do so because they view nurse–patient encounters as unique and it is this uniqueness that allows nurses to account for their work in terms of personal responsibility and not via some external standard or audit. However, that this approach necessarily involves a condemnation of the process of diagnosis – Ritter names Professor Ian Kennedy (1981) as someone who does this – is simply untrue. What concerns me, for instance, is the manner by which diagnoses are used as a green light for the kinds of subsequent care by which people, now seen as flawed, are progressively denied human rights. It is not about the correctness of biomedical constructs, it is about nurses aligning themselves with these such that their theoretical implications of flawed central nervous systems, for example, lead to a culture of inevitability and pessimism in the way that patients are related to. Hence, the importance of relationships where experience and intentionality have their place.

This is an issue of practice rather than theory but the problem with it is its resemblance to the basic civilities and moral requirements of everyday life. It does not lend itself to professionalism. By whatever means we evaluate relationships, be it through processes of 'being with', 'companionship' or 'truthfulness', these fail to identify the kinds of specific deficits which traditionally merit professional interventions. It is dissatisfaction with the essential ordinariness of nursing which leads to theoretical flights of fancy and notions of a fusion between the scientific and caring functions or that nurses will ultimately realise themselves by entering forms of mystical presence, uniting as one with their patients in a fusion of transpersonal existence. Even Kitson (1996: 1651) is prone to this kind of thinking: 'The future could hold the reconciliation of our two sides. It could herald the dawn of health care systems around the world committed to promoting health and well-being instead of systems that treat illness.'

Instead of? Are we to assume that treating illnesses is inappropriate? Of course, where Third World needs are dramatically different to those in the west, health care systems will achieve more by prevention. However, in addition to preventative measures, in Great Britain or America there remain the general tasks faced by illness treatment centres. It is a delusion to believe that economic, political or personal means can ensure health for all, and to believe that disease occurs because of some human omission (Kelly and Charlton 1995) when it often does not. The right to health becomes a moral imperative – and not a medical possibility – when it is converted to the idea that everyone can be healthy. Smail (1987) has no doubt that history and personal circumstances play a major role in human problems and he notes how the 'New Right' likes to foster the idea of personal responsibility for illness. When not doing that, it persuades psychiatric nurses that they should feel guilty for having looked after people who were not ill enough. However, whatever the complexities of economic or political systems in fostering illness and then providing for its treatment, the personal experience of illness cannot be ignored. Neither is it right for nurses to arbitrate on the seriousness of illness and whether or not to respond to it. In my view there is a moral dimension to nursing which requires that nurses respond to others irrespective of whether they have a viable therapy or not. There is much that is problematic in nursing if such responses are withheld on grounds of not possessing an evidence base by which to justify or argue one's actions. However, undue attention to the meaning of relationships in nursing can detract from the direct treatment of people's ills.

Responding to ill people with medical treatments is also to care; presumably doctors prescribe the best treatment because they think that it will work but also, ultimately, because they care. To nurse individuals, however, is arguably an ethically stronger event since not motivated by the anticipated success or other specific outcomes of treatments. Nurses perceive their status as a profession to be dependant on grounds of knowledge when their worth may be more highly evaluated in respect of its moral status. It is unfortunate that we live in a society which has difficulty accepting such a proposal and of finding ways of rewarding nurses accordingly.

References

1 Psychiatric nursing: illusion and reality

Andreasen, N.C. (1985) *The Broken Brain: The Biological Revolution in Psychiatry*, New York: Harper.

Baker, P. (1995) *The Voice Inside: A Practical Guide to Coping with Hearing Voices*, Manchester: Handsell Publications.

Bandler, R. and Grinder, J. (1979) *Frogs into Princes: Neurolinguistic Programming*, Moab, UT: Real People Press.

Barker, P.J. (1997) *Assessment in Psychiatric and Mental Health Nursing: In Search of the Whole Person*, Cheltenham: Stanley Thorne.

Barker, P., Reynolds, W. and Stevenson, C. (1998) 'The human science basis of psychiatric nursing: theory and practice', *Perspectives in Psychiatric Care* 34: 5–15.

Bowers, L. (1997) 'Commentary: the future of community psychiatric nursing', *Journal of Advanced Nursing* 4: 153–60.

Breggin, P. (1993) *Toxic Psychiatry*, London: Harper Collins.

Brooker, C. and Repper, J. (1998) *Serious Mental Health Problems in the Community: Policy, Practice and Research*, London: Bailliere Tindall.

Brooker, C. and White, E. (1990) *Community Psychiatric Nursing: A Research Perspective*, London: Chapman and Hall.

—— (1993) *Community Psychiatric Nursing: A Research Perspective*, vol. 2, London: Chapman and Hall.

—— (1995) *Community Psychiatric Nursing: A Research Perspective*, vol. 3, London: Chapman and Hall.

—— (1998) *The Fourth National Quinquennial Census of Community Mental Health Nursing*, Final Report to the Department of Health.

Caudill, W. (1958) *The Psychiatric Hospital as a Small Society*, Cambridge, MA: Harvard University Press.

Churchland, P.S. (1988) 'Reduction and the neurological basis of consciousness', in A.J. Marcel and E. Bisiach (eds) *Consciousness in Contemporary Science*, Oxford: Clarendon Press.

Clare, A. (1996) *In The Psychiatrist's Chair*, London: Kandarin Books.

Clarke, L. (1991) 'Ideological themes in mental health nursing', in P. Barker and S. Baldwin (eds) *Ethical Issues in Mental Health*, London: Chapman and Hall.

—— (1994) 'A further critical description of the therapeutic community', *Journal of Clinical Nursing* 3: 279–88.

—— (1996) 'Participant observation in a secure unit: care, conflict and control', *Nursing Times Research* 1: 431–40.

Clarke, L. and Whittaker, M. (1998) 'Self-mutilation: culture, contexts and nursing responses', *Journal of Clinical Nursing* 7: 129–37.

Clay, J. (1996) *R.D. Laing: A Divided Self*, London: Hodder & Stoughton.

Cole, A. (1997) 'The state we're in', *Nursing Times* 95: 24–7.

Cooper, D. (1970) *Psychiatry and Anti-Psychiatry*, London: Tavistock.

Crow, T.J. (1993) 'The search for a psychosis gene', *British Journal of Psychiatry* 158: 611–14.

Darcy, P. (1994) 'Accountability and the mental health services', *British Journal of Nursing* 3: 254–5.

Davis, B.D. (1981) 'Trends in psychiatric nursing research', *Nursing Times* 77: 73–6.

DSM IV (1994) *Diagnostic and Statistical Manual of Mental Disorder*, Washington: American Psychiatric Association.

Dudley, H.A.F. (1996) 'I believe...', *Proceedings of the Royal College of Physicians, Edinburgh* 26: 265–71.

Ellis, A. (1962) *Reason and Emotion in Psychotherapy*, New York: Lyle Stuart.

Gamble, C. (1995) 'The Thorn nurse training initiative', *Nursing Standard* 9: 31–4.

Gillam, T. (1995) 'Book review', *Nursing Times* 91: 49.

Glasser, W. (1975) *Reality Therapy: A New Approach to Psychiatry*, London: Harper & Row.

Gournay, K. (1995) 'Schizophrenia: a review of the contemporary literature and implications for mental health nursing theory, practice and education', *Journal of Psychiatric and Mental Health Nursing* 3: 7–12.

—— (1997) 'Responses to: what to do with nursing models – a reply from Gournay', *Journal of Psychiatric and Mental Health Nursing* 4: 227–31.

Gournay, K. and Beadsmore, A. (1995) 'The report of the clinical standards advisory group: standards of care for people with schizophrenia in the UK and implications for mental health nursing', *Journal of Mental Health and Psychiatric Nursing* 2: 359–64.

Gournay, K. and Brooking, J. (1994) 'Community psychiatric nurses in primary health care', *British Journal of Psychiatry* 165: 232–8.

Hanfling, O. (1978) *Uses and Abuses of Argument*, Milton Keynes: Open University Press.

Hart, C. (1994) *Behind the Mask: Nurses, their Unions and Nursing Policy,* London: Bailliere Tindall.

Henderson, D.K. and Gillespie, R.D. (1956) *A Textbook of Psychiatry*, Oxford: Oxford University Press.

Horrobin, D. (1980) 'A singular solution for schizophrenia', *New Scientist* 85 (1196): 642–4.

Jones, M. (1982) *The Process of Change*, London: Routledge.

Lloyd, G.E.R. (1970) *Hippocratic Writings*, Harmondsworth: Pelican.

Loach, K. (1971) *Family Life*, London: Woodfall Films.

Macdonald, V. and Merrit, M. (1996) 'Fish oil key to finding cure for schizophrenia', *The Daily Telegraph*, 15 September.

McFadyen, J.A. and Vincent, M. (1998) 'A reappraisal of community mental health nursing', *Mental Health Nursing* 18: 19–23.

Martin, J.P. (1984) *Hospitals in Trouble*, Oxford: Basil Blackwell.

Mason Cox, J. (1896) *Practical Observations on Insanity in which some Suggestions are Offered Towards an Improved Mode of Treating Diseases of the Mind to which are Subjoined Remarks on Medical Jurisprudence as Connected with Diseased Intellect*, 2nd edn, London: Baldwin & Murray.

May, D. and Kelly, M.P. (1982) 'Chancers, pests and poor wee souls: problems of legitimation in psychiatric nursing', *Sociology of Health and Illness* 4: 279–99.

Mental Health Nursing Review Team (1994) London: HMSO.

Morrall, P. (1994) 'Policing the mad', paper read at English National Board for Nursing and Midwifery Annual Conference (Mental Health), Ripon: Ripon College.

Mundt, C. and Spitzer, M. (1993) 'History of philosophy of mind and mental disorder', *Current Opinion in Psychiatry* 6: 704–8.

Nursing Times (July 1998) 94: 7.

Pembroke, L. (1991) 'Surviving psychiatry', *Nursing Times* 87: 30–2.

Pollock, L. (1989) *Community Psychiatric Nursing: Myth and Reality*, London: Scutari.

Rees, T.P. (1957) 'Back to moral treatment and community care', *Journal of Mental Science* 103: 303–13.

Richardson, J. (1998) 'One law for nurses, one law for consultants', *Nursing Times* 94: 18.

Ritter, S. (1997) 'Taking stock of psychiatric nursing', in S. Tilley (ed.) *The Mental Health Nurse: Views of Practice and Education*, Oxford: Blackwell Science.

Rogers, A. and Pilgrim, D. (1996) *Mental Health Policy in Britain: A Critical Introduction*, London: Macmillan.

Rose, S. (1998) 'The genetics of blame', *New Internationalist*, 20 April: 20–1.

Ross, L., Pollock, L. and Tilley, S. (1998) 'Community psychiatric nurse: what does it mean?' *Mental Health Nursing* 18 (1): 10–14.

Sakel, M. (1938) *The Pharmacological Shock Treatment of Schizophrenia*, Nervous and Mental Diseases Monograph Series no. 62, New York: Nervous and Mental Diseases Publishers.

Turgenev, I. (1965) *Fathers and Sons*, Harmondsworth: Penguin.

Ward, M. (1994) 'In search of a purpose', *Nursing Times* 90: 69.

Warner, L. (1997) 'Don't just role over and die', *Nursing Times* 93 (52): 30–1.

White, R. (1985) *Political Issues in Nursing: Past, Present and Future*, Chichester: John Wiley & Sons.

Wood, G. (1983) *The Myth of Neurosis: A Case for Moral Therapy*, London: Macmillan.

2 The whole truth?

Allen, C. (1990) 'P2000 problems', *Nursing Standard* 5 (6): 43–4.

Annual International Medical Review (1976) 84 (603/1).

Barker, P. (1995) *The Way Forward for Nurse Education*, address given 2 August at the English National Board Annual Conference (Mental Health), 31 July–2 October. Cambridge: Robinson College.

Baruch, G. and Treacher, A. (1978) *Psychiatry Observed*, London: Routledge & Kegan Paul.

Basford, L. and Slevin, O. (1995) *Theory and Practice of Nursing: An Integrated Approach to Patient Care*, Edinburgh: Campion.

Bjork, I.T. (1995) 'Neglected conflicts in the discipline of nursing: perceptions of the importance and value of practical skill', *Journal of Advanced Nursing* 22 (1): 6–12.

Blattner, B. (1981) *Holistic Nursing Care*, New York: Prentice Hall.

Chinn, P.L. (1987) 'Nursing theory development: where we have been and where we are going', in N. Chaska (ed.) *The Nursing Profession: A Time to Speak*, Toronto, Ont: McGraw-Hill.

Cloutier Laffrey, S. (1996) 'Community, culture, and truth in nursing inquiry', in J.F. Kikuchi, H. Simmons and D. Romyn (eds) *Truth in Nursing Inquiry*, London: Sage.

Cormack, D. (1983) *Psychiatric Nursing Described*, London: Churchill Livingstone.

Davidson-Rada, M. and Davidson-Rada, J. (1993) 'The rainbow model of health as ongoing transformation', *Journal of Holistic Nursing* 11 (1): 53.

Davies, E. and Lynch, S. (1995) 'Nursing: a rhythm of awakening', in G. Gray and R. Pratt (eds) *Scholarship in the Discipline of Nursing*, London: Churchill Livingstone.

Elliott, H. (1997) 'Holistic nursing and the therapeutic use of self', *Complementary Therapies in Nursing and Midwifery* 3: 81–2.

Engler, J.E. (1983) 'Buddhist Satipatthana-Vipassana meditation and an object relations model therapeutic development change: a clinical case study', unpublished dissertation: University of Chicago.

Farrell, B.A. (1981) *The Standing of Psychoanalysis*, Oxford: Oxford University Press.

Foot, P. (1967) *Theories of Ethics*, Oxford: Oxford University Press.

Fromm, E. (1978) *To Have or To Be?*, London: Abacus.

Gorman, J. (1995) *Openmind* 76: 19.

Gournay, G. (1995) 'Schizophrenia: a review of the contemporary literature and implications for mental health nursing theory, practice and education', *Journal of Psychiatric and Mental Health Nursing* 3: 7–12.

Graham, H. (1990) *Time, Energy and Psychology of Healing*, London: Jessica Kingsley.

Hale, W.R. (1997) 'Healing charisma in two kinds of healing communities', *Therapeutic Communities* 18 (1): 39–53.

Harris, M. (1995) 'Do nurses care for patients any more?', *Daily Mail*, 28 September.

Johnson, J.L. (1996) 'Nursing art and prescriptive truths', in A.F. Kikuchi, H. Simmons and D. Romyn (eds) *Truth in Nursing Inquiry*, London: Sage.

Jolley, M. and Brykcznska, G. (1992) *Nursing Care: The Challenge to Change*, London: Edward Arnold.

Kant, I. (1949) *Fundamental Principles of the Metaphysic of Morals*, trans. T.K. Abbott, Buffalo, New York: Prometheus.

Kennedy, I. (1981) *The Unmasking of Medicine*, London: Allen & Unwin.

Kikuchi, J.F. and Simmons, H. (1996) 'The whole truth', in J.F. Kikuchi, H. Simmons and D. Romyn (eds) *Truth in Nursing Inquiry*, London: Sage.

Kitson, A. (1988) 'On the concept of nursing care', in G. Fairbairn and S. Fairbairn (eds) *Ethics in Nursing Care*, Aldershot: Avebury.

Laing, R.D. (1965) *The Divided Self: An Existentialist Study in Sanity and Madness*, London: Penguin.

Liddle, P.F. (1994) 'The neurobiology of schizophrenia', *Current Opinion in Psychiatry* 7, 1: 43–6.

Macleod Clark, J., Maben, J. and Jones, K. (1996) *Project 2000: Perceptions of the Philosophy and Practice of Nursing*, London: English National Board for Nursing.

Malan, D. (1979) *Individual Psychotherapy and the Science of Psychodynamics*, London: Butterworth.

Morrison, P. (1997) 'The caring attitude in nursing practice: a repertory grid study of trained nurses' perceptions', *Nurse Education Today* 11: 3–12.

Neuman, B. (1989) *The Neuman Systems Model*, London: Prentice Hall.

North, M. (1972) *The Secular Priests*, London: George Allen & Unwin.

Owen, M.J. and Holmes, C.A. (1993) 'Holism in the discourse of nursing', *Journal of Advanced Nursing* 18: 1688–95.

Patterson, E.F. (1998) 'The philosophy and physics of holistic health care: spiritual healing as a workable interpretation', *Journal of Advanced Nursing* 27: 287–93.

Phillips, D.C. (1977) *Holistic Thought in Social Science*, London: Macmillan.

Pietroni, P.C. (1977) 'Holistic medicine', in A. Bullock, O. Stallybrass and S. Trombley (eds) *The Fontana Dictionary of Modern Thought*, London: Fontana.

Reed, J. and Ground, I. (1997) *Philosophy for Nursing*, London: Arnold.

Rew, L. (1996) 'The individual as a measure of truth', in J.F. Kikuchi, H. Simmons and D. Romyn (eds) *Truth in Nursing Inquiry*, London: Sage.

Russell, B. (1946) *History of Western Philosophy*, London: George Allen & Unwin.

Schober, J. (1995) 'Nursing: current issues and the patient's perspective', in *Towards Advanced Nursing Practice: Key Concepts for Health Care*, London: Arnold.

Scruton, R. (1995) *A Short History of Modern Philosophy: From Descartes to Wittgenstein*, London: Routledge.

Seedhouse, D. and Cribb, A. (1989) 'Introduction', in D. Seedhouse and A. Cribb (eds) *Changing Ideas in Health Care*, Chichester: John Wiley & Sons.

Smuts, J.C. (1926) *Holism and Evolution*, London: Macmillan.

Sokal, A. and Bricmont, J. (1998) *Intellectual Impostures: Postmodern Philosopher's Abuse of Science*, London: Profile.

Sunday Telegraph (1998) 'Letters Section: "Put nurses back on bedpan duty"', 15 February: 34.

Szasz, T. (1974) *The Myth of Mental Illness: Foundations of a Theory of Personal Conduct*, New York: Harper & Row.

Tynan, K. (1981) *Show People: Profiles in Entertainment*, London: Virgin.

Watson, J. (1985) *Nursing: The Philosophy and Science of Caring*, Colorado: Associated University Press.

Webb, C. (1992) 'What is nursing?', *British Journal of Nursing* 1: 567–8.

Williams, K. (1978) 'Ideologies of nursing: their meanings and implications', in R. Dingwall and J. McIntosh (eds) *Readings in the Sociology of Nursing*, Edinburgh: Churchill Livingstone.

3 Carl's world

Bradshaw, A. (1998) 'Defining "competency" in nursing (part II): an analytic review', *Journal of Clinical Nursing* 7: 103–111.

Brewster Smith, M. (1967) 'The phenomenological approach to personality theory: some critical remarks', in T. Millon (ed.) *Theories of Psychopathology*, London: W.B. Saunders Company.

Buber, M. (1937) *I and Thou*, Edinburgh: Clark.

Cohen, D. (1997) *Carl Rogers: A Critical Biography*, London: Constable.

Dalrymple, T. (1995) 'Don't bite the doctors', *The Sunday Times*, news section, 12 November: 3.

Dudley, H.A.F. (1996) 'I believe...', *Proceedings of the Royal College of Physicians, Edinburgh* 26: 265–71.

Freire, P. (1987) *A Pedagogy for Liberation: Dialogues on Transforming Education*, Basingstoke: Bergin and Macmillan.

Goffman, E. (1972) *Interaction Ritual: Essays on Face-to-Face Behaviour*, London: Allen Lane.

Halmos, P. (1965) *The Faith of the Counsellors*, London: Constable.

Hamlyn, D.W. (1987) *The Penguin History of Western Philosophy*, Harmondsworth: Penguin.

Heider, F. (1958) *The Psychology of Interpersonal Relations*, London: Wiley.

Husserl, E. (1964) *Ideas for a Pure Phenomenology*, trans. W.P. Alston and G. Nakhnikian, The Hague: Martinus Nijhoff.

Illich, I. (1975) *Medical Nemesis: The Expropriation of Health*, London: Calder & Boyars.

Kirchenbaum, H. (1979) *On Becoming Carl Rogers*, New York: Delacorte.

Kovel, J. (1978) *A Complete Guide to Therapy*, Harmondsworth: Penguin.

Maslow, A. (1987) *Motivation and Personality*, London: Harper & Row.

Masson, J. (1990) *Against Therapy*, London: Harper Collins.

Nye, R.D. (1992) *Three Psychologies: Perspectives from Freud, Skinner and Rogers*, 4th edn, Pacific Grove, CA: Brooks and Cole.

Pilgrim, D. (1997) *Psychotherapy and Society*, London: Sage.

Robbins Committee on Education (1963) *Report of the Committee appointed by the Prime Minister under the Chairmanship of Lord Robbins*, London: HMSO.

Rogers, C.R. (1951) *Client-centred Therapy: Its current Practice Implications and Theory*, London: Constable.

—— (1980) *A Way of Being*, Boston, MA: Houghton Mifflin.

Shanley, E. (1988) 'Inherently helpful people wanted', *Nursing Times* 84 (3): 34–5.

Tanner, M. (1994) *Nietzsche*, Oxford: Oxford University Press.

Thorne, B. (1992) *Carl Rogers*, London: Sage.

Walden, G. (1998) 'Her selflessness always got maximum publicity', *Evening Standard*, 17 April: 9.

4 Flowers in their mouths

Adler, R.B., Rosenfeld, L.B. and Towne, N. (1980) *Interplay: The Process of Interpersonal Communication*, New York: Holt, Rinehart & Winston.

Archbold, R. (1986) 'Ethical issues in qualitative research', in W.C. Chenitz and J.M. Swanson (eds) *From Practice to Grounded Theory: Qualitative Research in Nursing*, Massachusetts: Addison-Wesley.

Becker, H.S. and Geer, B.G. (1970) 'Participant observation and interviewing: a comparison', in R. Adams and J. Preiss (eds) *Human Organisation Research*, Illinois: Dorrey.

Bloor, M.J. (1980) 'The nature of therapeutic work in the therapeutic community – some preliminary findings', *International Journal of Therapeutic Communities* 1: 80–91.

Bluglass, R. (1978) 'Regional secure units and interim security for psychiatric patients', *British Medical Journal* 1: 489–93.

Burns, N. and Grove, S.K. (1987) *The Practice of Nursing Research: Conduct, Critique and Utilisation*, London: W.B. Saunders & Co.

Butler, R.A. (1974) 'Interim report of the committee on mentally abnormal offenders', London: Home Office and DHSS Cmnd. 5698.

—— (1975) 'Report of the committee on mentally abnormal offenders', London: Home Office and DHSS Cmnd. 6244.

Clark, D.H., Hooper, D.F. and Oram, E.G. (1962) 'Creating a therapeutic community in a psychiatric ward', *Human Relations* 15, 123–47.

Clarke, L. (1993) 'The opening of doors in British mental hospitals in the 1950s', *History of Psychiatry* 4: 527–51.

Clifford, C. and Gough, R. (1990) *Nursing Research: A Skills-Based Introduction*, London: Prentice Hall.

Cormack, D. (1981) 'Making use of unsolicited research data', *Journal of Advanced Nursing* 6: 41–9.

Evaneshko, V. (1985) 'Entree strategies for nursing field research studies', in M.M. Leininger (ed.) *Qualitative Research Methods in Nursing*, London: Grune & Stratton.

Fuller, J.R. (1985) 'Treatment environments in secure psychiatric settings: a case study', *International Journal of Offender Therapy and Comparative Criminology* 29 (1): 64–78.

Glancy, J.E. (1974) 'Revised report of the D.H.S.S. working party on security in NHS psychiatric hospitals', London: DHSS.

Goffman, E. (1959) *The Presentation of Self in Everyday Life*, Harmondsworth: Penguin.

—— (1961) *Asylums*, Harmondsworth: Penguin.

Gray, M. (1994) 'Data collection methods', in G. LoBiondo-Wood and J. Haber (eds) *Nursing Research: Methods, Critical Appraisal and Utilisation*, London: Mosby.

Grey, W.J. (1973) 'The therapeutic community and evaluation of results', *International Journal of Criminology and Penology* 1: 327–34.

Heller, J. (1974) *Something Happened*, London: Jonathan Cape.

Lofland, J. (1976) *Doing Social Life: The Qualitative Study of Human Interaction in Natural Settings*, New York: John Wiley & Sons.

Lofland, J. and Lofland, L.H. (1984) *Analysing Social Settings: A Guide to Qualitative Observation and Analysis*, California: Wadsworth.

May, D. and Kelly, M.P. (1982) 'Chancers, pests and poor wee souls: problems of legitimation in psychiatric nursing', *Sociology of Health and Illness* 4: 279–301.

Menzies, I. (1960) 'A case study in the functioning of social systems as a defence against anxiety', *Human Relations* 13: 95–121.

Morrison, V. (1983) 'Inarticulate speech of the heart', London: Mercury Records (March) 1983: MERL 16.

O'Brian, W.B. (1974) 'The Daytop Model for Addiction Treatment', paper presented to the Skandia International Symposium on Drug Dependence – Treatment and Treatment Evaluation, Stockholm, 17 October.

Olsen, V. and Whittaker, E. (1968) *The Silent Dialogue: A Study in the Social Psychology of Professional Socialisation*, San Francisco, CA: Jossey-Bass.

Pilgrim, D. and Eisenberg, N. (1985) 'Should special hospitals be phased out?', *Bulletin of the British Psychological Society* 38: 281–4.

Polit, D.E. and Hungler, B.P. (1993) *Essentials of Nursing Research: Methods, Appraisal and Utilisation*, Philadelphia, PA: J.B. Lippincott Company.

Ragucci, A. (1972) 'The ethnographic approach to nursing research', *Nursing Research* 21 (6): 485–90.

Reid, B. (1991) 'Developing and documenting a qualitative methodology', *Journal of Advanced Nursing* 16: 544–51.

Robinson, D. and McGregor Kettles, A. (1998) 'The lost vision of nursing', *Psychiatric Care* 5: 126–9.

Robinson, J. (1987) 'The relevance of research to the ward sister', *Journal of Advanced Nursing* 12: 421–9.

Rose, N. (1998) 'Living dangerously: risk-thinking and risk management in mental health care', *Mental Health Care* 11: 263–6.

Rosenhan, D.L. (1973) 'On being sane in insane places', *Science* 179: 250–8.

Rubá'iyát of Omar Khayyám (1900) trans. E. Fitzgerald, London: Methuen.

Schatzman, L. and Strauss, A.L. (1973) *Field Research: Strategies for a Natural Sociology*, Englewood Cliffs, NJ: Prentice Hall.

Sharp, V. (1975) *Social Control in the Therapeutic Community*, Farnborough: Saxon.

Snowden, P.R. (1983) 'The regional secure unit programme: a personal appraisal: the present state of play and future plans', *Bulletin of the Royal College of Psychiatrists* 7: 138–40.

West, W.G. (1980) 'Access to adolescent deviants and deviance', in W.B. Shaffir, R.A. Stebbins and A. Turowetz (eds) *Fieldwork Experience: Qualitative Approaches to Social Research*, New York: St Martin's Press.

5   Nursing and postmodernity: a logical alliance?

Adamson, B.J., Kenny, D.T. and Wilson-Barnett, J. (1995) 'The impact of perceived medical dominance on the workplace satisfaction of Australian and British nurses', *Journal of Advanced Nursing* 21: 172–83.

Amis, K. (1991) *Memoirs*, Harmondsworth: Penguin.

Barker, P. (1995) 'The way forward for nurse education', paper presented to the English National Board Mental Health Conference, *Partnerships for Care*, 2 August, Cambridge: Robinson College.

Baudrillard, J. (1988) *Selected Writings*, M. Poster (ed.), Cambridge: Polity Press.

—— (1993) *The Transparency of Evil*, London: Verso.

Bleasdale, A. (1995) *Jake's Progress*, episode 2, 19 October, London: Channel 4 Television.

Blom-Cooper, L. (1992) 'Report of the committee of inquiry into Ashworth hospital', London: HMSO.

Bourne, B., Eichler, U. and Herman, D. (1987) *Modernity and its Discontents*, Nottingham: Hobo Press.

Centore, F.E. (1991) *Being and Becoming: A Critique of Postmodernism*, New York: Greenwood Press.

Cooper, D. (1967) *Psychiatry and Anti-psychiatry*, London: Tavistock.

Crawford, P., Nolan, P. and Brown, B. (1995) 'Linguistic entrapment: medico-nursing biographies as fiction', *Journal of Advanced Nursing* 22: 1141–8.

Derrida, J. (1967) *Of Grammatology*, trans. G.C. Spivak, Baltimore, MA: John Hopkins University Press.

DHSS (1969) 'Report of the committee of inquiry into allegations of ill-treatment of patients and other irregularities at the Ely hospital Cardiff', London: HMSO Cmnd. 3795.

—— (1971) 'Report of the Farleigh hospital committee of inquiry', London: HMSO Cmnd. 4557.

—— (1972) 'Report of the committee of inquiry into Whittingham hospital', London: HMSO Cmnd. 4861.

—— (1974) 'Report of the committee of inquiry into South Ockendon hospital', London: HMSO.

Dzurec, L.C. (1994) 'Schizophrenic clients' experiences of power: using hermeneutic analysis', *Image: Journal of Nursing Scholarship* 26: 155–9.

Etzioni, A. (1960) 'Interpersonal and structural factors in the study of mental hospitals', *Psychiatry* 23: 13–22.

Foucault, M. (1971) *Madness and Civilisation: A History of Insanity in an Age of Reason*, London: Tavistock.

—— (1973) *The Birth of the Clinic*, London: Tavistock.

Fox, N. (1993) *Postmodernism, Sociology and Health*, Buckingham: The Open University Press.

Frankel, B. (1990) 'The cultural contradictions of postmodernity', in A. Milner, P. Thomson and C. Worth (eds) *Postmodern Conditions*, New York: Berg Publishers.

Geras, N. (1995) *Solidarity in the Conversation of Human Kind: The Ungroundable Liberalism of Richard Rorty*, London: Verso Press.

Guardian (1996) 'Nurse charged', news in brief section, 13 April: 4.

Harvey, D. (1992) 'The condition of postmodernity', in K. Thomson (ed.) *Modernity and its Futures*, Milton Keynes: Polity Press in association with the Open University.

Hewiston, A. (1995) 'Nurses' power in interaction with patients', *Journal of Advanced Nursing* 21: 75–82.

Holdsworth, N. (1997) 'Commentary: postmodernity and psychiatric nursing', *Journal of Psychiatric and Mental Health Nursing* 4: 309–12.

Ignatieff, M. (1987) 'Commentary', in B. Bourne, U. Eichler and D. Herman (eds) *Modernity and its Discontents*, Nottingham: Hobo Press.

Jacobs, E. (1995) *Kingsley Amis: A Biography*, London: Hodder & Stoughton.

Kelly, M.P. and Charlton, B. (1995) 'The modern and the postmodern in health promotion', in R. Bunton, S. Nettleton and R. Berrows (eds) *Sociology of Health Promotion*, London: Routledge.

Lacan, J. (1977) *Ecrits: A Selection*, trans. A. Sheriden, New York: W.W. Norton.

Laing, R.D. (1959) *The Divided Self*, Harmondsworth: Penguin Books.

Laing, R.D. and Esterson, A. (1964) *The Families of Schizophrenics*, London: Tavistock.

Lemon, M.C. (1995) *The Discipline of History and the History of Thought*, London: Routledge.

Lezzard, N. (1996) 'You cannot be serious', *The Sunday Times*, Section 10, 7 January: 12–13.

Lunder, R. (1987) 'Looking back in anger', *Nursing Times* 83: 49–50.

Lyotard, J.-F. (1984) *The Postmodern Condition*, trans. G. Bennington and B. Massumi, Manchester: Manchester University Press.

Marshall, B.K. (1992) *Teaching the Postmodern: Fiction and Theory*, New York: Routledge.

Martin, J.P. (1984) *Hospitals in Trouble*, London: Basil Blackwell.

Nursing Times (1997) 'This week', 93: 7.

Pejlert, A., Asplund, K. and Norberg, A. (1995) 'Stories about living in a hospital ward as narrated by schizophrenic patients', *Journal of Psychiatric and Mental Health Nursing* 2: 269–77.

Penhale, B. (1995) 'Recognising and dealing with the abuse of older people', *Nursing Times* 91: 26–7.

Peplau, H. (1952) *Interpersonal Relations in Nursing*, New York: G.P. Putnam's & Sons.

Reed, P.G. (1995) 'A treatise on nursing knowledge development for the 21st century: beyond postmodernism', *Advanced Nursing Science* 17: 70–84.

Robb, B. (1967) *Sans Everything: A Case to Answer*, London: Nelson.

Rogers, C. (1961) *On Becoming a Person*, London: Constable.

Rorty, R. (1980) *Philosophy and the Mirror of Nature*, Princeton, NJ: Princeton University Press.

Rowden, R. (1998) 'Shut that door', *Nursing Times* 94: 14–15.

Sedgwick, P. (1982) *Psychopolitics*, London: Pluto Press.

Sokal, A. and Bricmont, J. (1998) *Intellectual Impostures: Postmodern Philosopher's Abuse of Science*, London: Profile Books.

Sontag, S. (1983) *Illness as Metaphor*, Harmondsworth: Penguin Books.

Stein, L. (1978) 'The doctor-nurse game', in R. Dingwall and J. McIntosh (eds) *Readings in the Sociology of Nursing*, Edinburgh: Churchill Livingstone.

Stockwell, F. (1972) *The Unpopular Patient*, London: RCN Publications.

Towell, D. (1975) *Understanding Psychiatric Nursing*, London: RCN Publications.

Tynan, K. (1994) *Kenneth Tynan Letters*, London: Weidenfeld & Nicolson.

Vattimo, G. (1991) 'The end of (hi)story', in I. Hoesterey (ed.) *Zeitgeist in Babel: The Postmodernist Controversy*, Bloomington, IA: Indiana University Press.

Venturi, R. (1972) 'Mickey Mouse teaches the architect', *New York Times*, 22 October.

Vernon, M. (1995) 'A&E: why so complacent', *Nursing Times* 91: 28–30.

Watson, J. (1995) 'Postmodernism and knowledge development in nursing', *Nursing Science Quarterly* 8: 60–4.

Wilkinson, M.J. (1995) 'Love is not a marketable commodity: new public management in the British National Health Service', *Journal of Advanced Nursing* 21: 980–7.

Woolf, L. and Jackson, B. (1996) 'Coffee and condoms: the implementation of a sexual programme in acute psychiatry in an inner city area', *Journal of Advanced Nursing* 23: 299–304.

Wroe, M. (1995) 'Rave priest quits over sexual abuse', *The Observer*, news section, 28 November.

6 The socialisation of ideas in psychiatric nursing

Bannister, D. (1998) 'The nonsense of effectiveness', *Changes* 16: 21–30.

Baruch, G. and Treacher, A. (1978) *Psychiatry Observed*, London: Routledge & Kegan Paul.

Boyle, M. (1990) *Schizophrenia: A Scientific Delusion?*, London: Routledge.

Cohen, H.A. (1981) *The Nurses' Quest for a Professional Identity*, London: Addison-Wesley.

Firby, P.A. (1990) 'Nursing: a career of yesterday?', *Journal of Advanced Nursing* 15: 732–7.

Foucault, M. (1971) *Madness and Civilisation: A History of Insanity in an Age of Reason*, London: Tavistock.

Goodwin, S. and Mangan, P. (1985) 'Cosmic nursing: first step into the unknown', *Nursing Times* 81: 36–7.

Goodwin, S. and Mangan, P. (1990) 'The cosmic crusaders', *Nursing Times* 86: 28–9.

Gournay, K. (1995) 'Schizophrenia: a review of the contemporary literature and implications for mental health nursing theory, practice and education', *Journal of Psychiatric and Mental Health Nursing* 3: 7–12.

—— (1998) 'Face to face', *Nursing Times* 94: 40–1.

Gournay, K. and Grey, R. (1998) 'The role of new drugs in the treatment of schizophrenia', *Mental Health Nursing* 28: 21–4.

Hallstrom, C. (1998) 'Outside', *Mental Health Care* 1: 189.

Hickey, G. and Kipping, C. (1998) 'Who becomes a mental nurse?', *Nursing Times* 94: 53–5.

Ingleby, D. (1981) *Critical Psychiatry: The Politics of Mental Health*, Harmondsworth: Penguin.

Jaynes, J. (1976) *The Origins of Consciousness in the Breakdown of the Bicameral Mind*, Boston, MA: Houghton Mifflin.

Jenner, F.A., Monteiro, A.C.D., Zagalo-Cardoso, J.A. and Cunha-Oliviera, J.A. (1993) *Schizophrenia: A Disease or Some Ways of Being Human?*, Sheffield: Sheffield Academic Press.

Kavanagh, P. (1965) *Tarry Flynn*, London: Macgibbon & Kee.

Macleod Clark, J., Maben, K. and Jones, K. (1996) *Project 2000: Perceptions of the Philosophy and Practice of Nursing*, London: English National Board for Nursing and Midwifery.

Mason Cox, J. (1896) *Practical Observations on Insanity in which Some Suggestions are Offered Towards an Improved Mode of Treating Diseases of the Mind to which are Subjoined Remarks on Medical Jurisprudence as Connected with Diseased Intellect*, 2nd edn, London: Baldwin & Murray.

Melia, K. (1987) *Learning and Working: The Occupational Socialisation of Nurses*, London: Tavistock.

Morrall, P. (1994) 'Policing the mad', paper read at English National Board Annual (Mental Health) Conference, Ripon College.

Nietzsche, F. (1973) *Beyond Good and Evil: Prelude to a Philosophy of the Future*, Harmondsworth: Penguin.

Nursing Times (1998) 'Face to face', *Nursing Times* 94: 40–1.

Porter, R. (1987) *Mind Forg'd Manacles*, London: Athlone Press.

Ramon, S. (1985) *Psychiatry in Britain*, Beckenham: Croom Helm.

Sakel, M. (1938) *The Pharmacological Shock Treatment of Schizophrenia*, Nervous and Mental Diseases Monograph Series no. 62. New York: Nervous and Mental Diseases Publishers.

Sass, L.A. (1992) *Madness and Modernism: Insanity in the Light of Modern Art, Literature, and Thought*, London: Harvard University Press.

Spencer, A. (1994) 'The right choice', *Nursing Times* 90: 59–61.

Szasz, T. (1976) *The Myth of Mental Illness: Foundations of a Theory of Personal Conduct*, revised edn, London: Harper & Row.

—— (1994) *Cruel Compassion: Psychiatric Control of Society's Unwanted*, Chichester: Wiley.

Tilley, S. (1997) 'Introduction', in S. Tilley (ed.) *The Mental Health Nurse: Views of Practice and Education*, Oxford: Blackwell Science.

The Times (1998) 'NHS should use private firms to treat patients', 7 October: 12.

Warburton, N. (1992) *Philosophy: The Basics*, London: Routledge.

Williams, K. (1978) 'Ideologies of nursing: meanings and implications', in R. Dingwall and J. McIntosh (eds) *Readings in the Sociology of Nursing*, Edinburgh: Churchill Livingstone.

7 Ordinary miseries: extraordinary remedies

Bandler, R. and Grinder, J. (1990) *Frogs into Princes: Neurolinguistic Programming*, London: Eden Grove.

Baron, C. (1987) *Asylum into Anarchy*, London: Free Association Books.

Bergin, A. E. (1971) 'The evaluation of therapeutic outcomes', in A.E. Bergin and S.L. Garfield (eds) *Handbook of Psychotherapy and Behaviour Change*, New York: Wiley.

Bettelheim, B. (1983) *Freud and Man's Soul*, New York: Alfred A. Knopf.

Burnard, P. (1994) 'The emperor's new clones', *Nursing Standard* 8: 48–9.

Clare, A. (1981) *Let's Talk About Me*, London: BBC Publications.

Clarke, L. (1990) 'Rational Emotive Therapy', *British Journal of Psychotherapy* 7: 86–93.

—— (1993) 'Ordinary miseries: extraordinary remedies', *British Journal of Psychotherapy* 10: 237–48.

Clegg, P. (1995) 'Ethics and education in psychiatric nursing', in P. Martin (ed.) *Psychiatric Nursing*, London: Scutari Press.

Corney, R. (1988) 'Editorial', *Counselling: The Journal of the British Association for Counselling* 63: 1.

DHSS (1963) *Robbins Committee on Higher Education*, Cmnd. 2154, London: HMSO.

Dryden, W. (1990) *Rational Emotive Counselling in Action*, London: Sage.

Dryden, W. and Mearns, D. (1991) 'Rational-emotive therapy: a response', *British Journal of Psychotherapy* 7: 275–7.

Durlack, J. (1979) 'Comparative effectiveness of paraprofessional and professional helpers', *Psychological Bulletin* 86: 80–92.

Dye, N. (1995) 'My therapist sexually abused me', *More Magazine* 190: 62–4.

Egan, G. (1986) *The Skilled Helper: A Systematic Approach to Effective Helping*, Monterey, CA: Brooks/Cole Publishing.

Ellis, A. (1984) 'Must most psychotherapists remain as incompetent as they now are?', In J. Hariman (ed.) *Does Psychotherapy Really Help People?*, Springfield, IL: Charles J. Thomas.

Eysenck, H.J. (1985) *Decline and Fall of the Freudian Empire*, London: Viking.

Farrell, B.A. (1963) 'Psychoanalysis: the method', *New Society* 39: 12–13.

Fielding, R.G. and Llewelyn, S.P. (1987) 'Communication training in nursing may damage your health and enthusiasm: some warnings', *Journal of Advanced Nursing* 12: 281–90.

Garfinkel, H. (1967) *Studies in Ethnomethodology*, Englewood Cliffs: Prentice Hall Inc.

Gellner, E. (1985) *The Psychoanalytic Movement*, London: Paladin.

Hayek, F.A. (1978) *The Three Sources of Human Values*, L.T. Hobhouse Memorial Lecture 44, 17 March, London School of Economics Imprint: London.

Hersen, M. Michelson, L. and Bellack, S. (1984) *Issues in Psychotherapy Research*, New York: Plenum Press.

Jacobs, M. (1985) *The Presenting Past: An Introduction to Practical Psychodynamic Counselling*, Milton Keynes: Open University Press.

Kavanagh, P. (1970) 'Prelude', in B. Kennelly (ed.) *The Penguin Book of Irish Verse*, Harmondsworth: Penguin Books.

Lambert, M.J., Bergin, A.E. and Collins, J.L. (1977) 'Therapist induced deterioration in psychotherapy', in A.S. Gurman and A.Z. Razin (eds) *Effective Psychotherapy: A Handbook of Research*, New York: Pergamon Press.

LaTourette, A. (1987) 'The kindness of strangers', in D. Cohen (ed.) *The Power of Psychology*, Beckenham: Croom Helm.

Malan, D.H. (1979) *Individual Psychotherapy and the Science of Psychodynamics*, London: Butterworths.

Malcome, J. (1982) *Psychoanalysis: The Impossible Profession*, New York: Vintage Books.

Marks, I. (1977) *Nursing in Behavioural Psychotherapy: An Advanced Clinical Role for Nurses*, London: Royal College of Nursing Publication.

Masson, J. (1997) *Against Therapy*, London: Harper Collins.

Mearns, D. (1991) 'Response to Rational Emotive Therapy', *British Journal of Psychotherapy* 7: 275.

Medawar, P.R. (1975) 'Victims of psychiatry', *New York Review of Books*, 23 January.

Neuro-Linguistic Programming Brochure (1995), Pace Personal Development, 86, South Hill Park, London NW3 2SN.

Pinter, H. (1981) 'Notes from a programme for *The Birthday Party*', London: Tavistock Repertory Company.

Rogers, C.R. (1967) *On Becoming a Person: A Therapist's View of Psychotherapy*, London: Constable.

Rowan, J. (1994) 'Done it again', *British Journal of Psychotherapy* 10, 596–7.

Rycroft, C. (1968) *A Critical Dictionary of Psychoanalysis*, London: Nelson.

Shanley, E. (1988) 'Inherently helpful people wanted', *Nursing Times* 84: 34–5.

Smail, D. (1978) *Psychotherapy: A Personal Approach*, London: Dent.

Stern, M.H. (1972) *International Journal of Psychoanalysis* 53: 13.

Strupp, H. (1973) *Psychotherapy: Clinical Research and Clinical Issues*, New York: Jason Aronson.

Strupp, H.H., Hadley, S.W., Gomes, B. and Armstrong, S.H. (1976) 'Negative effects in psychotherapy: a review of clinical and theoretical issues with recommendations for a programme of research', report to the NIMH, Washington D.C.

Truax, C.B. (1966) 'Reinforcement and non-reinforcement in Rogerian psychotherapy', *Journal of Abnormal Psychology* 71: 1–9.

Truax, C.B. and Carkhuff, R. (1967) *Toward Effective Counselling and Psychotherapy*, Chicago, IL: Aldine.

Walker, M. (1990) *Women in Therapy and Counselling*, Milton Keynes: Open University Press.

Ward, M. (1995) 'Therapy as abuse', *Asylum*, Spring: 28–30.

Weldon, F. (1993) 'Will no one rid us of these turbulent priests?', *The Times*, Saturday Review, 20 February: 4–6.

Wootton, B. (1959) *Social Science and Social Pathology*, London: George Allen & Unwin.

8 Rational emotive therapy

Barker, P. (1998) 'Face to face', *Nursing Times* 94: 4.

Clare, A. (1981) *Let's Talk About Me*, London: BBC Publications.

Dryden, W. (1986) 'Correspondence', in *British Journal of Psychotherapy* 3: 192.

Ellis, A. (1994) *Reason and Emotion in Psychotherapy*, New York: Carol Publishing.

Gamble, C. (1995) 'The Thorn nurse training initiative', *Nursing Standard* 9: 31–4.

Hudson, L. (1967) *Contrary Imaginations: A Psychological Study of the English Schoolboy*, Harmondsworth: Penguin.

Kovel, J. (1978) *A Complete Guide to Therapy: From Psychoanalysis to Behaviour Modification*, Harmondsworth: Penguin.

Malcolme, J. (1982) *Psychoanalysis: The Impossible Profession*, London: Picador.

Maslow, A. (1968) *Towards a Psychology of Being*, London: Van Nostrand Reinhold.

Neenan, M. and Dryden, W. (1996) 'Rational emotive behaviour therapy', *Counselling*, November: 317–21.

North, M. (1972) *The Secular Priests*, London: George Allen & Unwin.

Tennov, D. (1975) *The Hazardous Cure*, Garden City, NY: Anchor Press.

9 1999: a nursing odyssey?

Abel-Smith, B. (1960) *A History of the Nursing Profession*, London: Heinemann.

Beardshaw, V. and Robinson, R. (1990) 'New for old? Prospects for nursing in the 1990s', *Research Report 8*, London: King's Fund Institute.

Bridges, J.M. (1990) 'Literature review on the images of the nurse and nursing media', *Journal of Advanced Nursing* 15: 850–4.

Burke, P. (1977) 'Whig Interpretation of History', in A. Bullock, O. Stallybrass and S. Trombley (eds) *The Fontana Dictionary of Modern Thought*, London: Fontana Press.

Butterfield, H. (1965) *The Whig Interpretation of History*, New York: W.W. Norton.

Caine, T., Smail, D.J., Wijesinghe, O.B.A. and Winter, D.A. (1982) *The Claybury Selection Battery Manual*, Windsor: NFER-Nelson.

Carpenter, M. (1988) *Working for Health: The History of the Confederation of Health Service Employees*, London: Lawrence & Wisehart.

Caudill, W. (1958) *The Psychiatric Hospital as a Small Society*, Cambridge, MA: Harvard University Press.

Clarke, L. (1989) 'The effects of training and social orientation on attitudes towards psychiatric treatments', *Journal of Advanced Nursing* 14: 485–93.

—— (1991) 'Attitudes and interests of students and applicants from two branches of the British nursing profession', *Journal of Advanced Nursing* 16: 213–23.

Clarke, L. (1996) 'Psychiatric nursing and Project 2000', *Journal of Advanced Nursing* 23: 420–1.

Council of Deans and Heads of UK University Faculties for Nursing, Midwifery and Health Visiting (1998) *Breaking the Boundaries*, London.

Davis, B.D. (1981) 'Trends in psychiatric nursing research', *Nursing Times* 77: 73–6.

Elkan, R. and Robinson, J. (1995) 'Project 2000: a review of published research', *Journal of Advanced Nursing* 22: 386–92.

Gournay, K. (1986) 'A pilot study of nurses' attitudes with relation to post basic training', in J. Brooking (ed.) *Readings in Psychiatric Nursing Research*, Chichester: John Wiley.

—— (1995) 'New facts on schizophrenia', *Nursing Times* 91: 32–3.

Hart, C. (1994) *Behind the Mask: Nurses, their Unions and Nursing Policy*, London: Bailliere Tindall.

Jay, P. (1979) 'Report of the committee of inquiry into mental handicap nursing and care', London: HMSO.

Jowett, S., Walton, I. and Payne, S. (1994) *Challenges and Change in Nurse Education: A Study of the Implementation of Project 2000*, London: National Foundation for Educational Research in England and Wales.

Kirk, S., Carlisle, C. and Luker, K. (1997) 'The implications of Project 2000 and the formation of links with higher education for the professional and academic needs of nurse teachers in the United Kingdom', *Journal of Advanced Nursing* 26: 1036–44.

Le Var, R.M.H. (1997a) 'Project 2000: a new preparation for practice – has policy been realised?', part 1, *Nurse Education Today* 17: 171–7.

—— (1997b) 'Project 2000: a new preparation for practice – has policy been realised?', part 2, *Nurse Education Today* 17: 263–73.

Maben, J. and Macleod Clark, J. (1998) 'Project 2000 diplomates' perceptions of their experiences of transition from student to staff nurse', *Journal of Clinical Nursing* 7: 145–53.

Macleod Clark, J., Maben, J. and Jones, K. (1996) *Project 2000: Perceptions of the Philosophy and Practice of Nursing*, London: English National Board for Nursing and Midwifery.

McIntegart, J. (1990) 'A dying breed?', *Nursing Times* 86: 72.

Mental Health Nursing Review Team (1994) *Working in Partnership: A Collaborative Approach to Care*, London: HMSO.

Menzies-Lyth, I. (1988) *Containing Anxiety in Institutions*, London: Free Association Books.

Mort, L. (1996) 'Critical of care', *Nursing Times* 92: 40–1.

NHS Health Service Circular (1998) National Service Frameworks (HSC 1998/074), London: Department of Health.

Nolan, P. (1993) *A History of Mental Health Nursing*, London: Chapman and Hall.

Nursing Times (1997) Anonymous, letters section, 93 (1): 19.

Payne, S., Jowett, S. and Walton, I. (1991) *Nurse Teachers in Project 2000: The Experience of Planning and Initial Implementation*, Slough: NFER.

Phillips, M. (1999) 'How the college girls destroyed nursing', *The Sunday Times* 10 January: 13.

Robbins Committee on Higher Education (1963) Cmnd. 2154, London: HMSO.

Robinson, J. (1991) 'Project 2000: the role of resistance in the process of professional growth', *Journal of Advanced Nursing* 16: 820–4.

Rogers, B. (1998) 'Probation period only adds to stress of project 2000', *Nursing Times* 94 (15): 19.

Ryan, D. (1989) *Project 1999: The Support Hierarchy as the Management Contribution to Project 2000*, discussion paper 4, University of Edinburgh: Department of Nursing Studies.

Shanley, E. (1981) 'Attitudes of hospital staff to mental illness', *Journal of Advanced Nursing* 6: 199–203.

United Kingdom Central Council (1986) *Project 2000: A New Preparation for Practice*, London: United Kingdom Central Council.

White, E., Riley, E., Davies, S. and Twinn, S. (1994) *A Detailed Study of the Relationships Between Teaching, Support, Supervision and Role Modelling for Students in Clinical Areas within the Context of Project 2000 Courses*, London: English National Board for Nursing and Health Visiting.

White, R. (1985) *Political Issues in Nursing: Past, Present and Future*, Chichester: John Wiley & Sons.

Williamson, J. (1998) 'Nursing grudges', *The Daily Telegraph*, letters section, 1 March: 32.

Wilson, G. (1975) *Manual for the Wilson–Patterson Attitude Inventory*, Windsor: NFER-Nelson.

10 The search for conclusions

Allen, C. (1990) 'PK2000 problems', *Nursing Standard* 5, 43–4.

Arendt, M. (1992) 'Caring as everydayness', *Journal of Holistic Nursing* 10 (4): 285–93.

Barker, P.J. and Davidson, B. (1998) 'Epilogue: the Heart of the Ethical Matter', in P. Barker and S. Davidson (eds) *Psychiatric Nursing Ethical Strife*, London: Arnold.

Barker, P.J., Reynolds, W. and Ward, T. (1995) 'The proper focus of nursing: a critique of the "caring" ideology', *International Journal of Nursing Studies* 32 (4): 386–97.

Barker, P., Reynolds, W. and Stevenson, C. (1998) 'The human science basis of psychiatric nursing', *Perspectives in Psychiatric Care* 34: 5–14.

Benner, P. (1984) *From Novice to Expert: Excellence and Power in Clinical Nursing Practice*, London: Addison-Wesley.

Bjork, I.T. (1995) 'Neglected conflicts in the discipline of nursing: perceptions of the importance and value of practical skill', *Journal of Advanced Nursing* 22: 6–12.

Blom-Cooper, L. (1992) 'Report of the Committee of Inquiry into Ashworth Hospital', London: HMSO.

BMA (1996) *Towards Tomorrow*, London: BMA.

Brecher, R. (1988) 'On not caring about the individual', in G. Fairbairn and S. Fairbairn (eds) *Ethical Issues in Caring*, Aldershot: Avebury.

—— (1995) personal communication.

Brooker, C. and Repper, J. (1998) *Serious Mental Health Problems in the Community*, London: Bailliere Tindall.

Brooker, C. and White, E. (1998) *The Fourth Quinquennial National Community Mental Health Nursing Census of England and Wales*, published jointly by the Universities of Manchester and Keele.

Brown, J.M., Kitson, A. and McKnight, T.J. (1992) *Challenges in Caring: Explorations in Nursing and Ethics*, London: Chapman and Hall.

Campbell, P. (1995) 'The service user's perspective on the care programme approach', English National Board Annual Conference (Mental Health) 1 August, Yorkshire: Ripon College.

Carr, P. (1984) 'Legal and ethical perspectives in the nursing care of the mentally ill', *Community Psychiatric Nursing Journal* 4: 14–18.

Clarke, L. (1991) 'Attitudes and interests of students and applicants from two branches of the British nursing profession', *Journal of Advanced Nursing* 16: 213–23.

Community Psychiatric Nursing Journal (1984–94).

Cormack, D. (1983) *Psychiatric Nursing Described*, Edinburgh: Churchill Livingstone.

Davidson, B. (1998) 'The role of the psychiatric nurse', in P. Barker and S. Davidson (eds) *Psychiatric Nursing Ethical Strife*, London: Arnold.

Davies, E. and Lynch, S. (1995) 'Nursing: a rhythm of human awakening', in G. Gray and R. Pratt (eds) *Scholarship in the Discipline of Nursing*, London: Churchill Livingstone.

Dawkins, R. (1998) *Unweaving the Rainbow*, London: Allen Lane, Penguin Press.

De Raeve, L. (1993) 'The nurse under physician authority: commentary', *Journal of Medical Ethics* 19: 228–9.

DHSS (1969) 'Report of the committee of inquiry into allegations of ill-treatment of patients and other irregularities at the Ely Hospital Cardiff', London: HMSO Cmnd. 3795.

DHSS (1971) 'Report of the Farleigh Hospital committee of inquiry', London: HMSO Cmnd. 4557.

DHSS (1972) 'Report of the committee of inquiry into Whittingham Hospital', London: HMSO Cmnd. 4861.

DHSS (1974) 'Report of the committee of inquiry into South Ockendon Hospital', London: HMSO.

Diels, D. (1994) 'Debate: what is nursing?', in J. McCloskey and H.K. Grace (eds) *Current Issues in Nursing*, London: Mosby.

DoH (1990) *Working in Partnership: A Collaborative Approach to Care*, Report of the Mental Health Nursing Review Team, London: HMSO.

Gournay, K. (1995) 'Schizophrenia: a review of the contemporary literature and implications for mental health nursing theory, practice and education', *Journal of Psychiatric and Mental Health Nursing* 3: 7–12.

Greer, G. (1973) 'Woman power', in J.A. Ogilvy (ed.) *Self and World: Readings in Philosophy*, New York: Harcourt Brace Jovanovich.

Gregory, R. (1997) *Eye and Brain: The Psychology of Seeing*, Oxford: Oxford University Press.

Harris, M. (1995) 'Do nurses care for patients any more?', *Daily Mail*, 28 September.

Holden, R.J. (1996) 'Nursing knowledge: the problem of the criterion', in J.F. Kikuchi, H. Simmons and D. Romyn (eds) *Truth in Nursing Inquiry*, London: Sage.

Hunt, G. (1994) 'Introduction: ethics, nursing and the metaphysics of procedure', in G. Hunt (ed.) *Ethical Issues in Nursing*, London: Routledge.

Johnson, J.L. (1996) 'Nursing art and prescriptive truths', in J.F. Kikuchi, H. Simmons and S. Romyn (eds) *Truth in Nursing Inquiry*, London: Sage.

Kelly, M.P. and Charlton, B. (1995) 'The modern and the postmodern in health promotion', in R. Bunton, S. Nettleton and R. Berrows (eds) *Sociology of Health Promotion*, London: Routledge.

Kennedy, I. (1981) *Unmasking Medicine* (The Reith Lectures 1980), London: BBC Publications.

Kitson, A. (1988) 'On the concept of caring in nursing', in G. Fairbairn and S. Fairbairn (eds) *Ethics in Nursing Care*, Aldershot: Avebury.

—— (1996) 'Does nursing have a future?', *British Medical Journal* 313: 1647–51.

—— (1997) 'Using evidence to demonstrate the value of nursing', *Nursing Standard* 11 (28): 34–9.

Lunder, R. (1987) 'Looking back in anger', *Nursing Times* 83: 49–50.

McFarlane, J. (1988) 'Nursing: a paradigm for caring', in G. Fairbairn and S. Fairbairn (eds) *Ethical Issues in Caring*, Aldershot: Avebury.

McKeown, T. and Lowe, C.R. (1974) *An Introduction to Social Medicine*, Oxford: Blackwell Scientific.

May, T. (1993) 'The nurse under physician authority', *Journal of Medical Ethics* 19: 223–7.

Mental Health Act (1959) London: HMSO.

Nightingale, F. (1952) *Notes on Nursing*, London: Gerald Duckworth & Co.

Nursing Times (1995) news section, 91: 5.

Orlando, I.J. (1961) *The Dynamic Nurse-Patient Relationship: Function, Processes and Principles*, New York: G.P. Putnam & Sons.

Parse, R. (1992) 'Human Becoming: Parse's Theory of Nursing', *Nursing Science Quarterly* 5: 35–42.

Peters, P. (1995) 'A vision of hospital hell', *The Sunday Telegraph*, 24 September.

Phillips, M. (1999) 'How the college girls destroyed nursing', *The Sunday Times*, 10 January.

Porter, R. (1996) 'Two cheers for psychiatry! The social history of mental disorder in twentieth century Britain', in H. Freeman and G. Berrios (eds) *150 Years of British Psychiatry*, vol. 2, *The Aftermath*, London: Athlone.

Ritter, S. (1997) 'Taking stock of psychiatric nursing', in S. Tilley (ed.) *The Mental Health Nurse: Views of Practice and Education*, Oxford: Blackwell Science.

Robb, B. (1967) *Sans Everything: A Case to Answer*, London: Nelson.

Rogers, C.R. (1980) *A Way of Being*, Boston, MA: Houghton Mifflin.

Salvage, J. (1985) *The Politics of Nursing*, London: Heinemann.

Schlotfeldt, R.M. (1996) 'Common sense, truth and nursing knowledge development', in J.K. Kikuchi, H.S. Simmons and D. Romyn (eds) *Truth in Nursing Inquiry*, London: Sage.

Sharma, T. (1992) 'Patient voices', *Health Services Journal* 16: 20–1.

Shotter, J. (1975) *Images of Man in Psychological Research*, London: Methuen.

Smail, D. (1987) *Taking Care: An Alternative to Therapy*, London: Dent.

Sourial, S. (1997) 'An analysis of caring', *Journal of Advanced Nursing* 26: 1189–92.

Stockwell, F. (1972) *The Unpopular Patient*, London: Royal College of Nursing.

—— (1985) *The Nursing Process in Psychiatric Nursing Care*, Beckenham: Croom Helm.

Studdy, S. (1999) 'This week', *Nursing Times* 95: 8.

Vernon, M. (1995) 'A&E: why so complacent', *Nursing Times* 91: 28–30.

Walby, S., Greenwell, J., Mackay, L. and Soothill, K. (1994) *Medicine and Nursing: Professions in a Changing Health Service*, London: Sage.

Walker, L. and Advant, K. (1995) *Strategies for Theory Construction in Nursing*, London: Appleton & Lange.

Watson, J. (1989) 'Watson's philosophy and theory of human caring', in J.P. Riehl-Sisca (ed.) *Conceptual Models for Nursing Practice*, Norwalk, CT: Appleton & Lange.

White, R. (1985) 'Political regulators in British nursing', in R. White (ed.) *Political Issues in Nursing*, vol. 1, Chichester: John Wiley.

Williams, K. (1978) 'Ideologies of nursing: meanings and implications', in R. Dingwall and J. McIntosh (eds) *Readings in the Sociology of Nursing*, Edinburgh: Churchill Livingstone.

Williamson, J. (1998) 'Nursing grudges', *The Daily Telegraph*, 1 March.

Index